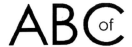

Diabetes

Seventh Edition

Tim Holt

Nuffield Department of Primary Care Health Sciences, Oxford University, UK

Sudhesh Kumar

Warwick Medical School, University of Warwick; and WISDEM, University Hospital, Coventry, UK

WILEY Blackwell

BMJ|Books

This edition first published 2015, © 2015 by John Wiley & Sons, Ltd
BMJ Books is an imprint of BMJ Publishing Group Limited, used under licence by John Wiley & Sons.

Registered Office
John Wiley & Sons, Ltd., The Atrium, Southern Gate, Chichester, West Sussex,
PO19 8SQ, UK

Editorial Offices
9600 Garsington Road, Oxford, OX4 2DQ, UK
The Atrium, Southern Gate, Chichester, West Sussex, PO19 8SQ, UK
111 River Street, Hoboken, NJ 07030-5774, USA

For details of our global editorial offices, for customer services and for information about how to apply for permission to reuse the
copyright material in this book please see our website at www.wiley.com/wiley-blackwell.

Library of Congress Cataloging-in-Publication Data

Holt, Tim A., author.
  ABC of diabetes / Tim Holt, Sudhesh Kumar. – Seventh edition.
    p. ; cm. – (ABC series)
  Includes bibliographical references.
  ISBN 978-1-118-85053-4 (pbk.)
I. Kumar, Sudhesh, author.   II. Title.   III. Series: ABC series (Malden, Mass.)
  [DNLM: 1. Diabetes Mellitus.   WK 810]
  RC660.4
  616.4′62–dc23

                          2015018781

A catalogue record for this book is available from the British Library.

Wiley also publishes its books in a variety of electronic formats. Some content that appears in print may not be available in electronic books.

Cover image: AlexRaths/Getty

Set in 9.25/11.5pt Minion by SPi Global, Pondicherry, India
Printed and bound in Singapore by Markono Print Media Pte Ltd

1   2015

Contents

Contributors to this Book

Aresh Anwar

Royal Perth Hospital, WA, Australia

Gurdev Deogon

Warwick Medical School, University of Warwick; and WISDEM, University Hospital, Coventry, UK

Tim Holt

Nuffield Department of Primary Care Health Sciences, Oxford University, UK

Noreen Kumar

St James's Hospital, Leeds, UK

Sudhesh Kumar

Warwick Medical School, University of Warwick; and WISDEM, University Hospital, Coventry, UK

Vinod Patel

Institute of Clinical Education, Warwick Medical School, Coventry; and George Eliot Hospital, Nuneaton, UK

Sailesh Sankar

WISDEM, University Hospital, Coventry and Warwickshire, Coventry, UK

Ponnusamy Saravanan

Clinical Sciences Research Institute, Warwick Medical School, Coventry; and George Eliot Hospital, Nuneaton, UK

Foreword

When I was a medical student in the late 1970s, diabetes was depicted to us as a disease of the pancreas, present in one per cent of the population and treated mostly in specialist centres by people called diabetologists. Type 1 diabetes was what young people had, and Type 2 was the kind you got when you were old. On my vascular firm, I clerked in a succession of diabetic patients (all smokers) who were booked for amputations. On my ophthalmology firm (in the days before systematic retinal screening), I regularly saw advanced, sight-destroying diabetic retinopathy. On my antenatal firm, I saw a stillborn infant delivered to a mother whose gestational diabetes had gone undiagnosed and (therefore) untreated.

What a long time ago that was!

These days, the prevalence of diabetes in the UK has risen to over 4% of the adult population, and Type 2 diabetes (a vascular disease as much as an endocrine one) occurs in schoolchildren, as well as in 'old' people. It is now managed mainly by the person with diabetes (remember that, as these authors rightly point out at the end of Chapter 3, 'for most of the time, people with diabetes are not ill'), supported by their primary health care team and with occasional input from specialists.

Advances in drug therapies, along with developments in the organisation and delivery of diabetes services (such as: nurse-led education; primary care based registration and surveillance; national programmes of retinal screening and smoking cessation support (together with a social trend of falling smoking rates); pro-active preconception and antenatal care; and fast-track referral services for acute problems), have made the ghastly, life-changing complications of diabetes extremely rare. People with diabetes now expect to live 'normal lives'. Some have ruled countries, made millions, been Bond Girls, swum the Channel or climbed Everest.

But despite its increasing 'normalisation' in contemporary society, diabetes remains a potential killer. It is still the commonest cause of blindness in the working population, and is a significant contributor to perinatal mortality statistics. Its prevalence is strongly patterned by both poverty and ethnicity. We now know beyond doubt that people with diabetes who do not receive systematic, structured, evidence-based and culturally congruent care will suffer avoidable harm, and may die a premature death.

As Julian Tudor Hart once said: 'Primary health care is doing simple things well, for large numbers of people, few of whom feel ill'. Nowhere is that maxim better illustrated than in community-based care of people with diabetes. The *ABC of Diabetes*, now in its 7th edition, offers clear and accessible summaries of both the evidence and the practicalities of diabetes care for the non-specialist.

Trish Greenhalgh
Professor of Primary Care Health Sciences
Oxford University

Preface

There are few challenges for health care providers greater than the rise in diabetes prevalence, a global phenomenon affecting populations throughout the world and sparing no sector of society. This expansion, often referred to as an 'epidemic', results not only from lifestyle choices and 'diabetogenic' environments, but also quite simply from increased life expectancy.

Improved life expectancy is, of course, a welcome and positive reflection of improving social conditions, nutrition, health care and education, particularly in developing countries, but it carries with it a risk to still under-resourced economies from the need for costly interventions related to diabetes complications. An example of this is the alarming rise in the need for renal replacement therapy (haemodialysis and renal transplantation) in people with diabetes now living long enough to require it. Even in well-resourced environments, this rise presents a huge health economic challenge, adding to the very significant human cost. Today's epidemic of diabetes is fuelled by the epidemic of obesity, and more effective management of obesity has a significant impact on diabetes. We have, therefore, included a chapter on obesity and its management in this 7th edition.

Long-term conditions tend to cluster within individuals, leading to the problems of complex co-morbidity and polypharmacy. Type 2 diabetes has become central to this phenomenon, first of all because it is more common among those rendered sedentary by long term musculoskeletal disorders and, also, because its presence has a substantial detrimental effect on the risk of cardiovascular events. This new edition includes revisions to the original chapters on managing co-morbid conditions with diabetes, as well as updated sections on the management of diabetes itself.

Throughout the past twenty years, the focus of delivery has shifted towards primary care for the majority of diabetes management. This book aims to equip primary care clinicians to handle this challenge, but it also includes chapters on hospital-based care of diabetic emergencies, as well as specialist areas such as retinopathy and kidney disease. Each individual practitioner needs to recognise their role and the limit of their expertise within the wider team. Coordination between primary and secondary care is vital to achieve effective and safe delivery of diabetes care in the population.

Modern health professionals are fortunate to have a wide range of effective interventions in their armament against the diabetes challenge, as well as unprecedented opportunities for integrated care through clinical software. In the chapters that follow, we will describe how these tools are most effectively applied to help the individuals that need them most; how we can, and should, avoid over-treatment as well as under-treatment; and how health care can best be organised to co-ordinate the efforts of the multidisciplinary team in partnership with patients and their families.

Tim Holt
Sudhesh Kumar

Acknowledgements

This book benefits from the advice and generous support of many of our colleagues across the UK, particularly at Warwick Medical School, University Hospital, Coventry, and Oxford University. While we take responsibility for the interpretation of current evidence in today's practice, we have been greatly assisted by the advice of others who have contributed to chapters, reviewed manuscript drafts and supported the process in other ways.

We would particularly like to thank our contributors, who have provided text, images, and updated advice. These are Dr Paul O'Hare, Dr Aresh Anwar, Dr Ponnusamy Saravanan, Dr Vinod Patel, Dr Sailesh Sankar (Consultant Physicians), Mr Gurdev Deogan (Senior Podiatrist), and Dr Noreen Kumar.

We are also indebted to Mr Gary Misson (consultant ophthalmologist), Professor Susan Jebb (professor of nutrition), Dr Roger Gadsby (Associate Clinical Professor), Wendy Goodwin (diabetes specialist nurse), Claire Holt (practice nurse), Mr Vinod Menon (consultant upper gastrointestinal Surgeon) and Alice Quayle (medical student).

We are grateful as always for the innumerable patients that we meet in everyday practice, who continue to deepen our understanding of diabetes and the ways that it affects everyday life. We hope that these insights have come through in the final manuscript.

Finally, we would like to thank the publishing team at Wiley-Blackwell for all their support, and Susan Watson for all her administrative assistance in the preparation of this book.

Tim Holt
Sudhesh Kumar

CHAPTER 1

Diagnosing Diabetes

Tim Holt[1] and Sudhesh Kumar[2]

[1]Nuffield Department of Primary Care Health Sciences, Oxford University, UK
[2]Warwick Medical School, University of Warwick; and WISDEM, University Hospital, Coventry, UK

OVERVIEW

- Diabetes produces a variety of clinical presentations, from acute to gradual onset.

- The diagnosis should be based on two separate tests, unless the patient is clearly symptomatic, in which case only one positive test is required.

- A combination of genetic and environmental factors contribute to the risk of diabetes.

- Impaired glucose regulation is an important risk factor, both for future diabetes and cardiovascular disease.

- Distinction between random and fasting samples is essential in interpreting the significance of borderline blood glucose levels.

Introduction

Diabetes mellitus is a common metabolic disorder that is defined by chronic hyperglycaemia. There are myriad underlying causes for the hyperglycaemia but, currently, much of our approach to treatment is empirical. Besides symptoms related to hyperglycaemia itself, such as thirst, polyuria and weight loss, it may also cause potentially life-threatening acute hyperglycaemic emergencies. It is a major cause of morbidity and premature mortality from long-term complications such as cardiovascular disease, blindness, renal failure, amputations and stroke. With good control of hyperglycaemia established early on, and continued life-long, an individual with diabetes can enjoy a good quality of life and reduce the risk of these long-term complications that are so detrimental to their life and wellbeing.

Prevalence of diabetes

In the United Kingdom, we have an estimated 2.9 million people with diabetes. The prevalence of both type 1 and type 2 diabetes is increasing. Type 2 diabetes is increasing far more rapidly, driven by increasing life expectancy and the epidemic of obesity. It is believed that there will be as many as 300 million people with diabetes worldwide by the year 2025. Most of this increase will occur in developing countries. The majority of children have insulin-requiring type 1 diabetes, while the vast majority of those aged over 25 years will have type 2 diabetes (Figure 1.1).

Types of diabetes

The types of diabetes have been classified by the WHO. Type 1 diabetes (previously referred to as insulin-dependent diabetes mellitus or IDDM) is due to absolute insulin deficiency and is usually an autoimmune disease, leading to the destruction of the insulin-secreting beta cells in the pancreas. In some cases, the cause of destruction of the beta cells is not known.

Type 2 (previously known as non-insulin dependent diabetes mellitus or NIDDM) results from relative insulin deficiency that may be associated with varying degrees of insulin action defects, known collectively as insulin resistance.

For a practising clinician, the implication of this diagnosis is that patients with type 1 diabetes require insulin straight away and insulin should not be stopped, as it is life-preserving. Type 2 patients can progress through several stages, and may require insulin later on in their disease.

Risk factors for diabetes

Genetics

Genetic susceptibility is important for both types of diabetes. Family history of type 1 diabetes, or other autoimmune diseases such as autoimmune thyroid disease, is associated with a higher risk of developing type 1 diabetes in the family. Inheritance in type 2 diabetes is far more complex, as there are many underlying causes. Furthermore, the risk varies according to the particular sub-type of type 2 diabetes. A family history of type 2 diabetes in a first degree relative is a strong risk factor for diabetes in that individual.

ABC of Diabetes, Seventh Edition. Tim Holt and Sudhesh Kumar.
© 2015 John Wiley & Sons, Ltd. Published 2015 by John Wiley & Sons, Ltd.

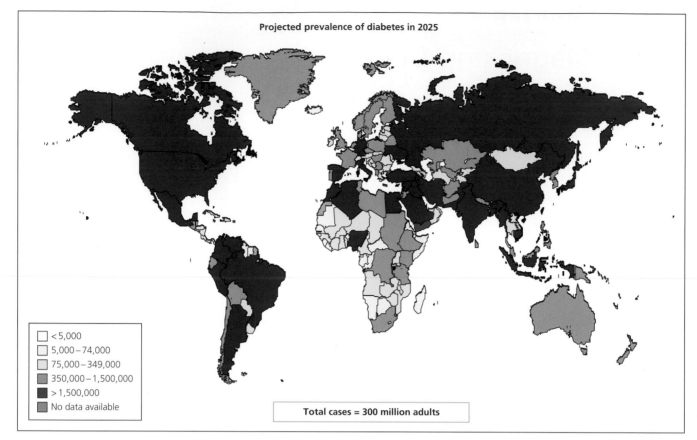

Projected prevalence of diabetes in 2025

Legend:
- < 5,000
- 5,000 – 74,000
- 75,000 – 349,000
- 350,000 – 1,500,000
- > 1,500,000
- No data available

Total cases = 300 million adults

Figure 1.1 Projected prevalence of diabetes in 2025. Source: World Health Organisation (1998). Reproduced with permission of World Health Organisation.

Obesity

Apart from family history, obesity is a very important risk factor for diabetes. For a given degree of obesity, central or 'apple-shaped' obesity is associated with a much higher risk of progression to type 2 diabetes than for those who have lower body obesity or are 'pear-shaped'. Those with a body mass index (BMI) of more than 25 kg/m² or high waist circumference (Table 1.1) are at a higher risk of developing diabetes, and they should be encouraged to take regular exercise and eat healthily (Figure 1.2).

Age

Beta cell function declines with age. Indeed, if we live long enough, all of us have the potential to develop diabetes at some stage. With an aging population, an increase in prevalence of diabetes can be expected.

Ethnicity

People of South Asian or Afro-Caribbean origin are at higher risk of developing diabetes. They are also more likely to have type 2 diabetes presenting at a young age, and usually have poorer risk factor control. South Asian patients have a high risk of developing diabetic renal disease and also coronary artery disease. Afro-Caribbean patients are more likely to have strokes, and have a higher risk of gestational diabetes. South Asian and Hispanic children may develop type 2 diabetes.

Table 1.1 The International Classification of adult underweight, overweight and obesity according to BMI (adapted from WHO guidelines, http://apps.who.int/bmi/index.jsp?introPage=intro_3.html).

Classification	BMI(kg/m²)	
	Principal cut-off points	Additional cut-off points
Underweight	<18.50	<18.50
Normal range	18.50–24.99	18.50–22.99
		23.00–24.99
Overweight	≥25.00	≥25.00
Pre-obese	25.00–29.99	25.00–27.49
		27.50–29.99
Obese	≥30.00	≥30.00
Obese class I	30.00–34.99	30.00–32.49
		32.50–34.99
Obese class II	35.00–39.99	35.00–37.49
		37.50–39.99
Obese class III	≥40.00	≥40.00

Source: Adapted from World Health Organisation 1995, 2000, 2004.

Initial presentation and diagnosis

The commonest presentation is tiredness, thirst, polyuria, weight loss, pruritus vulvae or balanitis. It is not uncommon for this diagnosis to be missed for years, and a significant proportion of those with type 2 diabetes remain undiagnosed. Insidious symptoms mean that the patients generally tend to ignore them. This is one

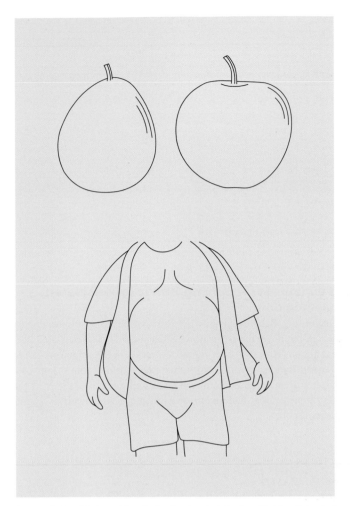

Figure 1.2 'Apple'-shaped fat distribution (central obesity with intra-abdominal adiposity) carries a higher cardiovascular and diabetes risk than 'pear'-shaped fat distribution.

Box 1.1 **Recommendation of the International Expert Committee**

For the diagnosis of diabetes:

- The HbA1c assay is an accurate, precise measure of chronic glycaemic levels and correlates well with the risk of diabetes complications.
- The HbA1c assay has several advantages over laboratory measures of glucose.
- Diabetes should be diagnosed when HbA1c is ≥ 48 mmol/mol. Diagnosis should be confirmed with a repeat HbA1c test. Confirmation is not required in symptomatic subjects with plasma glucose levels ≥ 11.1 mmol/l.
- If HbA1c testing is not possible, previously recommended diagnostic methods (e.g. FPG or two-hour OGTT, with confirmation) are acceptable.
- HbA1c should *not* be used to diagnose diabetes in certain circumstances, namely: pregnancy; children, young people or anyone following a type 1 presentation pattern; others in whom onset may be very recent, such as pancreatic injury; haemoglobin gene defects that affect red cell turnover and other causes of haemolysis.
- HbA1c testing may be indicated in children in whom diabetes is suspected but the classic symptoms and a casual plasma glucose ≥ 11.1 mmol/l are not found.

For the identification of those at high risk for diabetes:

- The risk for diabetes based on levels of glycemia is a continuum. Therefore, there is no lower glycemic threshold at which risk clearly begins.
- The categorical clinical states pre-diabetes, IFG and IGT fail to capture the continuum of risk, and they are being phased out of use as HbA1c measurements replace glucose measurements for diagnosis.
- Those with HbA1c levels below the threshold for diabetes, but ≥ 42 mmol/mol should receive demonstrably effective preventive interventions. Those with HbA1c below this range may still be at risk and, depending on the presence of other diabetes risk factors, may also benefit from prevention efforts.

Source: The International Expert Committee (2009).

reason why complications are often seen at diagnosis in patients with type 2 diabetes. A number of cases with type 2 diabetes are now diagnosed at insurance examinations, or through opportunistic testing, when the patient has presented for some other problem to the general practice or hospital.

The diagnosis of diabetes must not be taken lightly by a clinician, as the consequences for the individual are significant and life-long. For those presenting with severe symptoms, evidence of long-term complications or severe hyperglycaemia at presentation, the diagnosis is quite straightforward and can be made using only one diagnostic blood glucose or HbA1c measurement. In asymptomatic individuals presenting with mild hyperglycaemia, the diagnosis should only be established on the basis of at least two abnormal test results. One may use either glucose or HbA1c testing for diagnosis of diabetes (Box 1.1).

Glucose tolerance test

A glucose tolerance test should be performed in the morning after an overnight fast. It is important that the patient should have had a normal diet for the preceding three days and should not restrict carbohydrate intake drastically. The test should also not be performed during an acute illness or following prolonged bed rest. Plasma glucose concentrations are measured fasting, and then two hours after a drink of 75 g of glucose in 250–350 ml of water (in children: 1.75 g/kg, up to maximum of 75 g). Several proprietary preparations are available, and these are often flavoured to make items palatable.

Table 1.2 shows normal values and interpretation of abnormal values during an oral glucose tolerance test (OGTT). The role of oral glucose tolerance tests is changing, given the recommendations over the use of HbA1c as a preferred means of diagnosing diabetes (Box 1.1). It is still useful in those for whom HbA1c testing is inappropriate.

Table 1.2 WHO criteria for the diagnosis of diabetes mellitus based on venous plasma samples.

	Fasting (mmol/l)	Two-hour sample following oral glucose challenge (mmol/l) in OGTT
Normal	< 6.1	< 7.8
Impaired fasting glycaemia (IFG)	6.1–6.9	< 7.8
Impaired glucose tolerance (IGT)	< 7.0	7.8–11.0
Diabetes mellitus	≥ 7.0	≥ 11.1

Interpretation of the oral glucose tolerance test results

Impaired fasting glycaemia (IGF)

Fasting glucose between 6.1 and 6.9 mmol/l in the absence of abnormal values after the glucose load is defined as impaired fasting glycaemia. Conversion to diabetes is not invariable but it is important to reassess once a year, and in future this is likely to be through HbA1c measurement (see Box 1.1). Individuals with IFG should be advised about a healthy life-style and to avoid obesity.

Impaired glucose tolerance (IGT)

Once again conversion to diabetes is not invariable and patients may either persist with impaired glucose tolerance, revert to normal glucose tolerance or progress to type 2 diabetes. Obese individuals should be advised to try and lose weight through diet and exercise. The implications of this diagnosis for pregnancy are different, and this is considered further in Chapter 18.

IGF and IGT are collectively known as *impaired glucose regulation*. HbA1c has become the recommended means of diagnosing diabetes and identifying those at risk in the majority of patients (see Box 1.1). HbA1c levels of 42–47 mmol/mol are borderline and should trigger the same approach to prevention of diabetes and cardiovascular disease as the finding of IFG and IGT.

Diabetes mellitus

A fasting glucose of greater than or equal to 7.0 mmol/l or a two-hour glucose value of greater than or equal to 11.1 mmol/l suggests diabetes but, in future, this will be based on HbA1c (Box 1.1). The glucose tolerance test does not indicate the type of diabetes; this is usually determined on the basis of other presenting features, and is discussed further below. Young age at presentation (especially less than 17 years), presence of other autoimmune endocrine diseases (such as hypothyroidism, pernicious anaemia, Addison's disease, vitiligo) in the patient or family members, or significant weight loss, are features that suggest type 1 diabetes.

Diabetes in children

Abnormal blood glucose readings in a child or adolescent up to the age of 17 years should be taken seriously, as they may have type 1 diabetes. It is important to avoid delay in treatment, especially when they present with very high blood glucose levels. In those with mild hyperglycaemia, or where there is doubt, HbA1c should be measured (see Box 1.1).

Table 1.3 Conversion of DCCT aligned HbA1c measurements to the new IFCC standard.

HbA1c	
DCCT aligned (%)	IFCC (mmol/mol)
4	20
5	31
6	42
6.5	48
7	53
7.5	59
8	64
9	75
10	86
11	97
12	108

New units for reporting HbA1c (glycosylated haemoglobin)

Diagnosing diabetes has in the past been based on blood glucose values, but the diagnosis is now usually based on glycosylated haemoglobin (HbA1c). The measurement of HbA1c has required standardisation of reporting across the world. Table 1.3 gives a chart for converting the older DCCT-aligned units (%) to the new International Federation of Clinical Chemistry (IFCC) units (mmol/mol).

Identifying patients in need of insulin or urgent referral to hospital

Insulin is life-saving in those with type 1 diabetes, and is also indicated in all patients with marked hyperglycaemia or significant weight loss, particularly if ketosis is detected in the urine or blood. Children are much more likely to have type 1 diabetes. Any form of hyperglycaemia in pregnancy is also an indication for insulin. Patients who fail to achieve adequate glycaemic control on oral agents should also be given insulin. A patient who is unable to eat and drink normally, and has marked hyperglycaemia due to a concomitant illness, will require insulin and may need to be seen in hospital urgently.

Metabolic syndrome

Type 2 diabetes, hypertension, dyslipidaemia and central obesity often present in the same individual. This clustering of chronic risk factors has been called the metabolic syndrome. Therefore, the presence of central obesity, hypertension or dyslipidaemia should prompt the clinician to look for diabetes. It should be noted that the majority of patients with metabolic syndrome do not yet have overt type 2 diabetes, but may have either undiagnosed diabetes or impaired glucose tolerance. It is here that the concept of metabolic syndrome is particularly useful. As patients with diabetes should have other cardiovascular risk factors treated intensively anyway, identifying metabolic syndrome in such patients may not alter management.

Delaying the onset of type 2 diabetes

In those identified as being 'at risk', lifestyle changes to increase physical activity and a diet with modest calorie restriction, less saturated fat and more dietary fibre can significantly reduce the rate at which impaired glucose tolerance progresses to type 2 diabetes. It has been demonstrated that even older people can successfully undertake the lifestyle programmes required. This is discussed in more detail in Chapter 4.

Further reading and references

DECODE Study Group (2003). Is the current definition for diabetes relevant to mortality risk from all causes and cardiovascular and non-cardiovascular diseases? *Diabetes Care* **26**, 688–696.

Freemantle N, Holmes J, Hockey A, Kumar S (2008). How strong is the association between abdominal obesity and the incidence of type 2 diabetes? *International Journal of Clinical Practice* **62**, 1391–1396.

The International Expert Committee (2009). International Expert Committee Report on the role of the HbA1c assay in the diagnosis of diabetes. *Diabetes Care* **32**, 1327–1334.

World Health Organisation (1998). *The World Health Report. Life in the 21st Century: a vision for all*. Geneva: WHO.

World Health Organization (1999). *Definition, Diagnosis and Classification of Diabetes Mellitus and its Complications:* Report of a WHO Consultation. World Health Organization, Geneva. WHO/NCD/NCS 99.2.

CHAPTER 2

Types of Diabetes

Tim Holt[1] and Sudhesh Kumar[2]

[1]Nuffield Department of Primary Care Health Sciences, Oxford University, UK
[2]Warwick Medical School, University of Warwick; and WISDEM, University Hospital, Coventry, UK

OVERVIEW

- A number of different pathological mechanisms produce chronic hyperglycaemia, the hallmark of clinical diabetes.
- These mechanisms produce different patterns of presentation and, therefore, different types of diabetes.
- Important pathways include autoimmune destruction of beta cells in type 1 diabetes, and insulin resistance with gradual decline in beta cell function in type 2.
- Diabetes may also result from drug therapy or from systemic disease affecting other organs as well as the pancreas.
- There is increasing interest in the classification of sub-types of diabetes, which is assisting in the personalisation of treatments for affected individuals.

Introduction

Diabetes mellitus is not one disease. It is defined as chronic hyperglycaemia that may be caused by one or more of numerous underlying processes. Some of these cause diabetes directly, by interfering with beta cell function or through significant defects in insulin action. In other cases, diabetes is part of a more general disorder affecting many other organs or systems. Examples include: some endocrinopathies; drug- or chemical-induced diabetes; diabetes related to certain infections; and diabetes associated with certain genetic syndromes.

Although one might argue that management of diabetes is empirical, and that knowledge of the underlying causes does not alter management for most patients, this is changing. For some distinct sub-types of diabetes, there are clinical implications for patients and their families. In the future, this is likely to lead to increasing personalisation of drug therapy.

Type 1 diabetes

Type 1 diabetes results from destruction of the beta cells in the islet cells of Langerhans in the pancreas (Figure 2.1). This usually results in more or less absolute deficiency of insulin. In most cases, this is due to autoimmune destruction of the islets, resulting from a combination of genetic susceptibility and poorly understood environmental triggers that initiate the disease process. It is believed that this process starts a long time before the illness actually presents. There is, therefore, an opportunity for prevention of diabetes in the future, in this group of patients. Type 1 diabetes is far more common in those with a history of other autoimmune disorders, such as coeliac disease, thyroid disease, pernicious anaemia and Addison's disease. If there is a strong family history of any of these disorders, the risk of type 1 diabetes in these families is higher.

Genetic factors predisposing to type 1 diabetes

The strong concordance of type 1 diabetes in monozygotic twins suggests a major role for genetic factors. The major histocompatibility complex antigens are thought to be important. Most type 1 patients show either DR3 or DR4, while DR2 is thought to be protective against diabetes.

Autoantibodies in type 1 diabetes

Islet cell autoantibodies are present at diagnosis, but will gradually decline and disappear in ensuing years. This means that, if there is diagnostic uncertainty, islet cell antibodies can be checked early during presentation. Specific tests have been devised recently, including anti-GAD (glutamate decarboxylase) antibodies and also islet antibody-2 (IA-2) antibodies. The presence of both together is associated with a significantly higher risk of developing type 1 diabetes. The inclusion of a third antibody, anti-insulin antibody, will improve detection of Type 1 diabetes to nearly 100%.

ABC of Diabetes, Seventh Edition. Tim Holt and Sudhesh Kumar.
© 2015 John Wiley & Sons, Ltd. Published 2015 by John Wiley & Sons, Ltd.

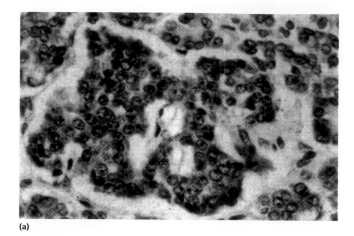

(a)

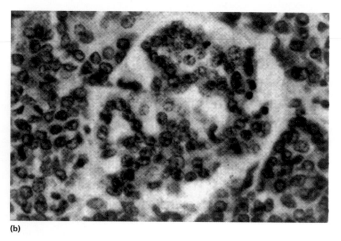

(b)

Figure 2.1 Beta cell destruction after 50 years of type 1 diabetes.

The use of these tests in clinical practice is restricted to situations where there is doubt about the diagnosis of the type of diabetes, and to distinguish from type 2 diabetes. Clinically, the implication is that if the tests are negative, the patient might then not require insulin. Attempts to prevent type 1 diabetes in these susceptible individuals have, thus far, not proved successful.

Type 2 diabetes

Type 2 diabetes is a complex heterogeneous condition, and recent genetic studies have revealed numerous sub-types. Children presenting with mild hyperglycaemia present diagnostic problems, as they may have latent slowly progressing type 1 diabetes. These children may then progress to requiring insulin. On the other hand, with increasing prevalence of obesity, more children are now presenting with type 2 diabetes, particularly those from ethnic minorities. In the USA, in some areas, up to 50% of children with diabetes are now presenting with the type 2 form.

Latent autoimmune diabetes in adults (LADA) is thought to comprise about 5% of all patients with type 2 diabetes. These people

have autoantibodies usually seen in type 1 diabetes, but their clinical presentation is like someone with type 2 diabetes. This is a group that may present an excellent opportunity for subsequent prevention of diabetes if an effective intervention can be developed to prevent further beta cell destruction.

Maternally inherited diabetes with deafness (MIDD)

This is a form of diabetes due to mutations in mitochondria, most commonly related to 3243A > G mitochondrial DNA mutation. Mitochondria in an individual are inherited from the mother, rather than from the father, so one clue would be evidence of strong maternal transmission of diabetes, particularly when this is associated with sensorineural deafness. Some patients may also have peripheral vision problems, particularly night blindness. These patients often require insulin.

Special forms of diabetes

Genetic sub-types of diabetes

Some sub-types of diabetes are now known to be important, as management will be different from the standard paradigm. For example, patients with a form of Maturity Onset Diabetes in the Young (MODY) due to HNF-1α (hepatocyte nuclear factor 1α) gene mutation are very sensitive to sulphonyureas, but metformin is less effective in these patients.

Monogenic diabetes is the term used for a collection of conditions that cause diabetes now shown to result from single gene defects. One feature of these conditions is that they show autosomal-dominant inheritance patterns, where the disease appears to be vertically transmitted (e.g. through several generations). It is also diagnosed before the age of 25 years but, unlike type 1 diabetes patients, monogenic diabetes patients do not often require insulin for at least five years after diagnosis.

Genetic testing in these cases can confirm the particular sub-type of diabetes. This can have significant clinical implications. Patients with HNF1α mutations, for example, exhibit exquisite sensitivity to sulphonylureas and can be successfully treated with tablets. Knowledge of the mutation, therefore, can help in the management of this disorder, even in children who would otherwise have been put onto insulin. This is also one form of type 2 diabetes where we would use a sulphonylurea in preference to metformin when initiating therapy.

Patients with HNF1β have renal cysts. Patients with glucokinase mutations are less common, but the diagnosis is significant for individuals and their families. Such patients are much less likely to develop complications of diabetes, because they mainly have mild fasting hyperglycaemia without significant post-meal hyperglycaemia.

Steroid-induced diabetes

A number of chronic inflammatory diseases are treated with glucocorticoids, and this is a cause of hyperglycaemia or unmasking of diabetes earlier in these patients. The main mechanism for

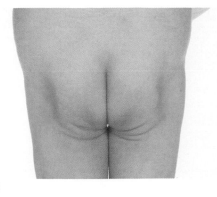
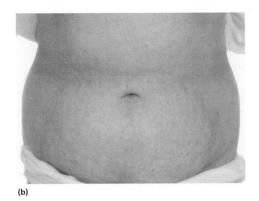

(a)   (b)

Figure 2.2 Lipodystrophy affecting the buttocks **(a)** but not the abdomen **(b)**.

diabetes in these patients is through inhibition of insulin secretion, and it is important to try and reduce the need for steroids in these patients. Clinically it is useful to remember that metformin is less useful in the management of this type of diabetes, and also that fasting glucose is not useful for diagnosis unless there is marked hyperglycaemia.

Ketosis prone diabetes

There are patients who present similar to type 2 diabetes until there is a major stress, such as an infection, when they may become either hyperglycaemic with ketosis or have frank diabetic ketoacidosis. Such patients may be able to withdraw insulin when they are well, and they do not show classical autoantibodies seen in Type 1 diabetes

Latent Autoimmune Diabetes in Adults (LADA)

This type of diabetes refers to adults who develop diabetes with many of the features suggestive of type 1 diabetes, with some features suggesting type 2 diabetes, yet they appear to be relatively stable without any need for insulin to preserve life. The confusion here is with type 1 diabetes, and it is also useful to recognise this group of patients because:

a they may need insulin sooner than other type 2 diabetic patients;
b there may be other autoimmune disorders in the same patient that needs screening for;
c in future there may be therapies that may be able to prevent progression to frank type 1 diabetes.

Lipodystrophies

It has been known for a long time that marked defects in adipose tissue distribution may be associated with diabetes. For example, complete absence of subcutaneous adipose tissue, as in generalised lipodystrophy or partial lipodystrophies with absence of fat in the face and torso, are associated with diabetes and dyslipidaemia. However, more recently, a much more common disorder

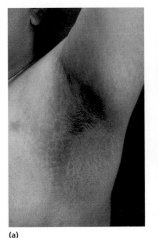
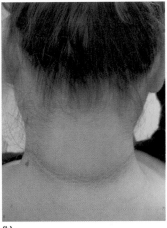

(a)   (b)

Figure 2.3 Acanthosis nigricans in the axilla **(a)** and behind the neck **(b)**.

of adipose tissue distribution, familial face-sparing lipodystrophy, has been recognised. These patients often have excess fat on the face, neck, abdomen and also visceral fat. They show marked lack of fat in the gluteal area and in the limbs (Figure 2.2). Often, patients also have acanthosis nigricans, seen particularly in the axilla or the back of the neck (Figure 2.3). These patients present with an insulin-resistant diabetes, often with hypertriglyceridaemia. Marked hypertriglyceridaemia can be a risk factor for pancreatitis, and should be managed with a low-fat diet and lipid-lowering medication.

Other insulin-resistant syndromes

Other rarer causes of insulin-resistant syndromes may present in childhood, with failure to thrive, growth problems and also acanthosis nigricans. Paradoxically, these children may exhibit fasting hypoglycaemia and yet, once they develop diabetes, may require large doses of insulin to control hyperglycaemia. If such disorders are suspected, referral to a specialist will be required, as the management can be quite difficult.

Further reading

Jafar-Mohammadi B, McCarthy MI (2007). Genetics of type 2 diabetes mellitus and obesity – a review. *Annals of Medicine* **18**, 1–9.

Lindgren CM, McCarthy MI (2008). Mechanisms of disease: genetic insights into the etiology of type 2 diabetes and obesity. *Nature Clinical Practice Endocrinology & Metabolism* **4**, 156–163.

Murphy R, Ellard S, Hattersley AT (2008). Clinical implications of a molecular genetic classification of monogenic beta-cell diabetes. *Nature Clinical Practice Endocrinology & Metabolism* **4**, 200–213. Review.

CHAPTER 3

Helping People Live with Diabetes

Tim Holt[1] and Sudhesh Kumar[2]

[1]Nuffield Department of Primary Care Health Sciences, Oxford University, UK
[2]Warwick Medical School, University of Warwick; and WISDEM, University Hospital, Coventry, UK

OVERVIEW

- Patient-centred priority setting and supported self-management form the modern approach to diabetes care.
- Targets should be tailored to the individual's needs and priorities.
- Patients are more likely to adhere to treatment plans that they have formulated themselves.
- Self-efficacy and 'ownership' of the condition should be nurtured through structured education.

Introduction

Living with diabetes is a long personal journey. Throughout the journey, patients require information, education, support and self-management skills. They also require prescribed medication, monitoring, surveillance and regular review. This journey is a joint venture between the individual, their carers and a multidisciplinary team of health professionals (Box 3.1).

Patient-centred priority setting

In the past, patients were expected to follow the doctor's instructions passively. Those who failed to reach targets were simply not complying. This approach was never very effective in diabetes, but it is increasingly insufficient in the modern world of patient autonomy, access to information and personal responsibility for health. We now know that individuals are much more likely to adhere to decisions that they have formulated themselves. The emphasis of diabetes care should be self-management, supported by a team of health professionals (Figure 3.1).

Shared decision-making

The Autonomous Patient: Ending paternalism in medical care by Angela Coulter (2002) suggests three models of clinical decision-making (Table 3.1).

The shared decision-making model is well established in primary care, where patients are usually not acutely ill. The clinician must provide and share information, while the patient must be prepared to discuss personal values and preferences. Both accept shared responsibility for the treatment decisions. A successful clinician-patient relationship, built on mutual trust, allows the model to be adapted flexibly to the situation. Development of a serious acute illness might shift the emphasis towards professional choice, while the need to choose a hospital for non-urgent cataract surgery might be purely a consumer choice.

Targets

Treatment targets should be tailored to different patient types, depending on co-morbidity, life expectancy, risk of hypoglycaemia, patient preferences, and other factors. Discussing personalised goals with the patient and sharing responsibility for keeping within targets is an important step in the successful control of risk factors (Box 3.2).

There is increasing awareness of the need for less stringent blood glucose control targets for older patients, particularly those at greater risk of cardiovascular disease (see Chapter 6). The benefits of tight glycaemic control are most evident for microvascular complications over relatively long timescales, while the macrovascular risk factors (blood pressure, lipids, smoking, obesity, physical inactivity) cause more immediate problems, through raising risk of myocardial infarction and stroke.

This should not prevent us from aiming for good control of blood glucose, which may improve quality of life through reduction in symptoms, particularly if such control can be achieved without drugs that risk hypoglycaemia (sulphonylureas, 'glinides', and insulin). It simply means that a further reduction towards truly 'normal' blood glucose levels carries a risk that may not be justified in older type 2 patients with diabetes of long duration and with co-morbidities. For those at diagnosis, however, tighter glycaemic control as part of a multifactorial approach should confer better long term outcomes, including preservation of renal function.

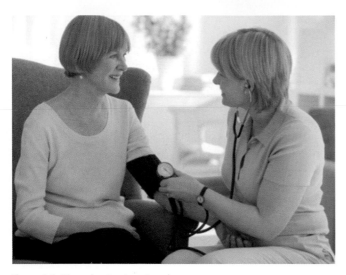

Figure 3.1 Discussing treatment goals.

Table 3.1 Models of clinical decision-making.

Professional choice	Shared decision making	Consumer choice
Clinician decides, patient consents	Information shared, both decide together	Clinician informs, patient makes decision

Source: Coulter (2002). Reproduced with permission of Nuffield Trust.

Tighter glycaemic control is generally appropriate for type 1 patients, who are usually younger at diagnosis and, therefore, have many years left to benefit from reduced development of microvascular disease, such as retinopathy and nephropathy. This does, however, depend on hypo risk and hypo awareness. Tight control is important if at all possible in pregnant patients, in view of the impact on both maternal and foetal outcomes (see Chapter 18). This is why individualised control targets are so important (Box 3.3).

It is generally recommended to control total serum cholesterol to ≤ 4.0 mmol/l and LDL cholesterol to ≤ 2.0 mmol/l. This is

Table 3.2 Type 2 diabetes – meeting the needs.

Readily achieved	Difficult to achieve
Blood pressure control	Durable control of glycaemia
Lipid management	Post-prandial glucose levels
Screening for complications	Abdominal obesity
Glycaemic control in early stages of disease	Smoking cessation
	Physical inactivity

particularly important in type 2 patients with established cardiovascular disease or risk factors for it. In practice, this includes the majority with type 2 diabetes (see Chapter 6).

Realistic weight reduction targets should be negotiated. Gradual, sustainable weight loss is far more beneficial than sudden loss, which is initially encouraging but then demoralising when the weight returns. The same applies to physical activity, which should gradually be increased to a moderate level over a period of time.

Some targets are easier to achieve than others (Table 3.2). Controlling blood pressure and lipids is usually possible, provided the individual concords with prescribed drug therapy. The more difficult areas are those requiring self-management skills and lifestyle change. It is now recognised that ongoing support (e.g. from commercial weight loss programmes) makes sustained weight reduction more likely, as individuals benefit not only from the advice but also from regular review, monitoring and encouragement.

Main issues to cover in the first consultation

- The biochemical basis for diabetes in lay terms (raised blood sugar, insufficient insulin, body not responding to insulin properly).

Box 3.4 **Lifestyle Changes and Drug Therapy**

Lifestyle change is important for the majority of patients, but some may feel disinclined to change their behaviour if they are immediately prescribed drug therapy. A period of behavioural adaptation following diagnosis before drugs are commenced may be beneficial unless the indication is strong. Three months is the traditional interval.

Box 3.5 **Self-efficacy**

'Self-efficacy' is a key element to the success of behavioural change in diabetes. The term refers to the individual's personal ability to take action and make changes. Self-efficacy is the basis for a number of diabetes management interventions, including DAFNE, DESMOND and the Diabetes Manual.

- Diabetes can cause problems with a number of organs and body systems, which can be prevented through a joint effort between the patient and the practice team.
- Controlling blood glucose levels reduces the chances of complications of diabetes, but controlling blood pressure and cholesterol are equally important.
- The importance of lifestyle, weight control and exercise not only reduce blood glucose, blood pressure, and cholesterol, but also make the body's own insulin work more effectively.
- Realistically, over time there is a tendency for the glucose levels to rise further, so that medication usually needs to be 'stepped up' as time goes by, even in a patient who 'does everything right'. It is important that patients do not feel demoralised by such an escalation (Box 3.4).
- Mention in outline the range of treatments – lifestyle change, tablets, insulin. Discuss insulin in a positive way (even though not needed now), and not as a 'last desperate resort'. This will help in future if the time comes when it is needed.
- Refer to 'lifestyle' or 'dietary' changes, rather than to 'dieting', to avoid patients believing that their treatment will involve a strict 'crash' diet that they are unlikely to sustain.

Keeping on the same side

Newly diagnosed patients sometimes feel overwhelmed at the prospect of self-managing a complex and potentially serious medical condition. Such individuals need structured education, support and confidence building, provided by a consistent and integrated team of health professionals. Developing our patients' knowledge and skills towards a state of self-efficacy (Box 3.5) is one of the most valuable things we can offer them in the early stages of diabetes.

Armande, the character played by Judi Dench in the 2000 film *Chocolat*, conceals her insulin-dependent diabetes at the local chocolaterie (Figure 3.2). Defying pressure from her daughter to enter institutional care, she follows the village's general slide into temptation, and dies through overindulgence in chocolate. Set in rural France in 1959, the story reflects the shifting social trend towards freedom of choice, and her death is portrayed as a victory for personal autonomy. But the basis for her defiance is a lack of self-efficacy, and the absence of a non-judgemental clinician she can trust. Adult patients rarely opt for the rebellion route if given sufficient support and a feeling of ownership of their condition.

How can we help patients change their lifestyles?

- Engage with the patient from the time of diagnosis.
- Be clearly 'on the same side'.
- Reinforce positive moves to change and praise achievements, even small ones.

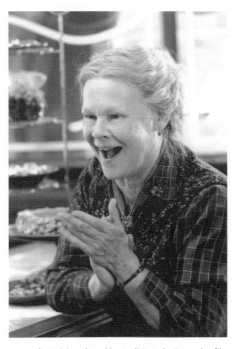

Figure 3.2 Armande Voizin, played by Judi Dench. From the film *Chocolat*. Photo credit: David Appleby/Courtesy of Miramax Film Corp.

Box 3.6 **Tools for Use in a Consultation**

- Use open questions.
- Listen to answers.
- Acknowledge beliefs and feelings.
- Be non-judgemental.
- Reflect and paraphrase.
- Help the patient to define an action plan and set timescales.

- Give consistent, supportive messages from all members of the team, using written material.
- Encourage the patient to access educational resources themselves, including reliable websites that support the same messages as the health team.
- Take it a little at a time and set realistic short-term goals.
- Emphasise the need to *maintain* change, which is more difficult than achieving it in the first place.
- Provide the actual figures: most patients can easily understand the basic indices and targets and, by feeling a sense of 'ownership' of the data, will accept responsibility for them (Box 3.6).

Structured education

As well as regular input from the practice team, patients may benefit from entering a structured education programme. This is particularly valuable following diagnosis, but it can be offered at any time. In the UK, available programmes include DESMOND and The Diabetes Manual (for type 2 patients) and DAFNE for type 1 patients.

- **DESMOND** (Diabetes Education and Self-Management for Ongoing and Newly Diagnosed) is an educational package to help people with type 2 diabetes, particularly those who are newly diagnosed. It has been shown to have benefits on weight loss and smoking cessation, and positive improvements in beliefs about illness. All aspects of self-management are covered, in a group setting.
- **The Diabetes Manual** is also designed for type 2 patients, but involves one-to-one education and is, therefore, suitable for those who prefer to avoid group education settings. In addition to a comprehensive manual, audiotapes are provided, and practice nurses are trained to deliver the educational material.
- **DAFNE** (Dose Adjustment For Normal Eating) is a five-day training programme for people with type 1 diabetes. It involves learning accurate carbohydrate counting and adjustment of insulin doses according to need. It is suitable for well-motivated patients whose diabetes is less than adequately controlled, who have been diagnosed for at least six months, and who are prepared to monitor four to six times a day and inject frequently, using a basal bolus regimen. It is based on the idea that tailoring insulin doses to the person's usual diet (which is, in principle, unrestricted) is the best way of achieving glycaemic control without increased hypoglycaemia. It has been shown in a randomised controlled trial to improve HbA1c levels (as well as quality of life scores) without increasing the frequency of severe hypoglycaemia.

'Yo-yoing'

There is a thriving market for faddish diets and alternative dietary advice, which should be resisted. Patients are understandably attracted to media publicity or anecdotal accounts of rapid weight loss, but such approaches are rarely sustainable, and 'yo-yoing' (fluctuating weight with no overall trend towards reduction) is much less likely to produce long-term health benefit than a sustainable approach. Yo-yoing is less likely if newly diagnosed patients are presented with a positive image of healthy food, rather than a simple list of prohibited items. Interest in food needs to be redirected, rather than extinguished. Offering a wide range of healthy options in a positive way will avoid the impression of a gastronomic prison sentence. See Chapter 11 for dietary advice for diabetes.

Semantics

Although many do not object to the term 'diabetic', a proportion finds it stigmatising. The term, when referring to an individual, has been 'banned' from many of the major publications, including the *British Medical Journal*. Its use as an adjective (e.g. 'the diabetic foot') is generally considered acceptable, but it should no longer be used as a noun. The same has occurred for people with epilepsy. The term 'patient' is appropriate in context, but we should not forget that, for most of the time, people with diabetes are not ill.

Summary

Modern diabetes care needs to be patient-centred, recognising that people are, on the whole, more likely to succeed in achieving targets if they themselves have formulated, or helped to formulate, the management plan. Care should also be individually tailored, while maintaining standards that are common to all patients. Confidence-building to promote self-efficacy, and keeping on the same side, are important, and deserve the necessary time commitment, particularly in the early stages after the diagnosis.

Further reading and references

Coulter A (2002). *The Autonomous Patient: Ending paternalism in medical care*. The Nuffield Trust. The Stationary Office, London.

DAFNE Study Group (2002). Training in flexible, intensive insulin management to enable dietary freedom in people with type 1 diabetes: dose adjustment for normal eating (DAFNE) randomised controlled trial. *British Medical Journal* **325**, 746.

Davies MJ, Heller S, Skinner TC *et al.* (2008). Diabetes Education and Self Management for Ongoing and Newly Diagnosed Collaborative. Effectiveness of the diabetes education and self management for ongoing and newly diagnosed (DESMOND) programme for people with newly diagnosed type 2 diabetes: cluster randomised controlled trial. *British Medical Journal* **336** (7642), 491–495.

Sturt J, Taylor H, Docherty A *et al.* (2006). A psychological approach to providing self-management education for people with type 2 diabetes: the Diabetes Manual. *BMC Family Practice* **7**, 70.

Tattersall R (2002). The expert patient: A new approach to chronic disease management for the twenty-first century. *Clinical Medicine Journal of the Royal College of Physicians of London* **2**, 227–229.

CHAPTER 4

Early Detection and Prevention of Diabetes

Tim Holt[1] and Sudhesh Kumar[2]

[1] Nuffield Department of Primary Care Health Sciences, Oxford University, UK
[2] Warwick Medical School, University of Warwick; and WISDEM, University Hospital, Coventry, UK

OVERVIEW

- Hyperglycaemia is among the top five determinants of worldwide mortality.
- Increasing life expectancy is the main driver of the global diabetes 'epidemic'.
- Increasing obesity and physical inactivity add to this effect, producing rising prevalence of type 2 diabetes in younger people.
- Prevention and early detection of diabetes are essential to offset the associated morbidity and mortality.
- Diabetes may be prevented by lifestyle interventions.
- Those at risk of type 2 diabetes are also at risk of cardiovascular disease and represent a large population with unmet health needs.

Introduction

Two hundred and fifty million people worldwide have diabetes, and 80% of these are likely to die of cardiovascular disease. The escalating prevalence is often referred to as an 'epidemic' but, unlike an infectious disease, which typically burns itself out after a time, there is no suggestion that this will happen to the global diabetes problem. Figure 4.1 shows the projected increase in estimated numbers of people with diabetes in different regions of the world by 2030, and the trend by age band in developed and developing countries.

Changes in population demography

Expansion of the over-65 population, occurring most rapidly in developing countries, is the single most important factor driving this trend, and rising obesity prevalence will only add to these estimates. Countries experiencing industrialisation are likely to witness the greatest increase in patient numbers and, in many of these areas, health care provision is under-developed.

Type 2 diabetes in the young

Meanwhile, in developed countries, a different phenomenon is occurring – the increasing recognition of type 2 diabetes in adolescents and young adults. This rise is largely linked to obesity. In the USA, this problem disproportionately affects African-American and Hispanic populations (Cali and Caprio, 2008; see Figure 4.2).

Increasing obesity prevalence, particularly in industrialised nations, results largely from behavioural rather than genetic factors. High-calorie foods containing simple carbohydrate and saturated fat, together with increasingly sedentary lifestyle patterns, have fuelled this trend. This problem must be addressed at all levels – individual choice, clinician advice and public health measures – in order to influence the food industry.

Impacting on the diabetes epidemic

Improved nutrition, environmental conditions and medical care, all extending life expectancy to age bands where diabetes is more prevalent, are driving the epidemic. The solution must come through early detection and intervention through preventive measures. This means not only reducing progression to diabetes, but also targeting groups at risk of diabetes for multifactorial cardiovascular risk reduction.

Pre-diabetes and macrovascular disease

Microvascular complications of diabetes are related to duration and severity of raised blood glucose. There is a much weaker relationship between hyperglycaemia and macrovascular complications, which may have been brewing for years before the onset of diabetes itself. Macrovascular disease is associated with insulin resistance, which may pre-date beta cell insufficiency and overt hyperglycaemia by decades, but is typically accompanied by hypertension and dyslipidaemia. This has raised interest in this early phase, and the concept of 'pre-diabetes', as much of the morbidity

---

ABC of Diabetes, Seventh Edition. Tim Holt and Sudhesh Kumar.
© 2015 John Wiley & Sons, Ltd. Published 2015 by John Wiley & Sons, Ltd.

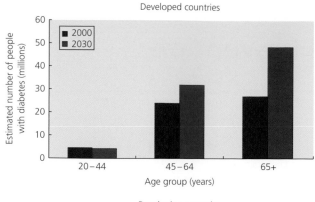

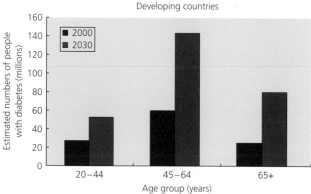

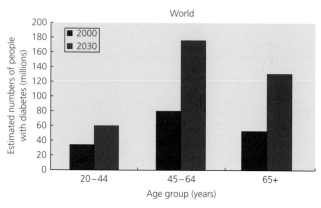

Figure 4.1 Projected numbers of people (thousands) with diabetes from 2000 to 2030 by region, and overall global rise in prevalence by age band. Source: Wild (2004). Reproduced with permission of American Diabetes Association.

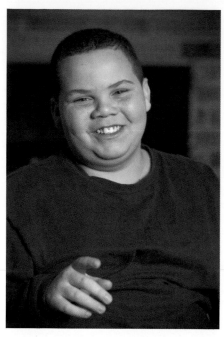

Figure 4.2 Childhood obesity is increasing the prevalence of type 2 diabetes in young people.

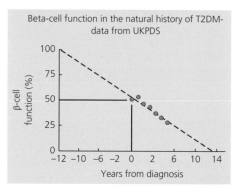

Figure 4.3 Beta cell function in the natural history of T2DM – data from UKPDS. Source: Holman (1998). Reproduced with permission of Elsevier.

Table 4.1 Relative risk of ischaemic heart disease and stroke for 1 mmol/l increase in fasting plasma glucose, by age group (after adjustment for confounding and regression dilution bias).

	<60 years	**60–69 years**	**≥70 years**
Ischaemic heart disease	1.424	1.196	1.196
Stroke	1.360	1.284	1.081

Source: Danaei *et al.* (2006). Reproduced with permission of Elsevier.

associated with it, is preventable. Beta cell function itself declines progressively prior to the diagnosis of diabetes (Figure 4.3).

The annual worldwide mortality associated with 'higher than optimal blood glucose levels' (which includes diabetes and the less severe borderline states) may be three times higher than that of diabetes itself (Danaei *et al.* 2006). This is because the numbers affected by these borderline levels is substantially greater than that of the diabetes population. The cardiovascular risk rises with increasing glycaemia from a level well below the threshold used to diagnose diabetes (Table 4.1). This puts raised blood glucose, whether or not high enough to be called diabetes, among the five top determinants of worldwide mortality, accounting for 3.16 million deaths a year (Diabetes Prevention Program Research Group, 2002; Figure 4.4).

The tip of the iceberg

In industrialised societies, and increasingly in the developing world, for every person in the community with diabetes there are many with the metabolic syndrome (Box 4.1) or other forms of 'pre-diabetes'. A quarter of the world's adults are estimated to have the metabolic syndrome, as defined by the International Diabetes

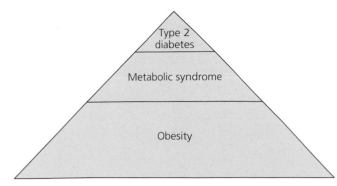

Figure 4.4 The 'iceberg' of preventable cardiovascular risk.

Box 4.1 The Metabolic Syndrome

Type 2 diabetes is a complex metabolic disorder, lying at one end of a spectrum of progressively impaired glucose regulation, insulin resistance and beta cell insufficiency. Central obesity, hypertension and dyslipidaemia usually accompany this constellation and, together, represent the 'metabolic syndrome'. Identifying this condition gives us an opportunity to delay the onset of diabetes and control the other cardiovascular risk factors that are part of the syndrome.

Box 4.2 The Metabolic Syndrome: International Diabetes Federation Definition

Central obesity (see Table 4.2) plus any two of the following four factors:

- Raised Triglyceride level: ≥ 1.7 mmol/l, or specific treatment for this lipid abnormality.
- Reduced HDL cholesterol: < 40 mg/dl (1.03 mmol/l*) in males and < 50 mg/dl (1.29 mmol/l*) in females, or specific treatment for this lipid abnormality.
- Raised blood pressure: systolic BP ≥ 130 or diastolic BP ≥ 85 mm Hg, or treatment of previously diagnosed hypertension.
- Raised fasting plasma glucose ≥ 5.6 mmol/l, or previously diagnosed type 2 diabetes.

*If above 5.6 mmol/l, an oral glucose tolerance test is strongly recommended but is not necessary to define the presence of the syndrome.

Federation (see Box 4.2). Such people have a 20% risk of developing diabetes. While many are currently living in the economically developed nations, less industrialised countries are developing similar lifestyle patterns and catching up.

Silent damage

Type 2 diabetes tends to develop gradually over long periods of time. Complications may be established, or even advanced, at the time of diagnosis. These affected up to 50% of newly diagnosed type 2 patients in the UKPDS Study. Macrovascular complications

Table 4.2 Ethnicity-specific definition of central obesity.

Country/Ethnic group		Waist circumference
Europids		
In the USA, the ATP III values (102 cm male; 88 cm female) are likely to continue to be used for clinical purposes	Male	≥94 cm
	Female	≥80 cm
South Asians, Chinese and Japanese		
Based on a Chinese, Malay and Asian Indian population	Male	≥90 cm
	Female	≥80 cm
Ethnic South and Central Americans	Use South Asian recommendations until more specific data are available	
Sub-Saharan Africans	Use European data until more specific data are available	
Eastern Mediterranean and Middle East (Arab) populations	Use European data until more specific data are available	

If BMI is > 30 kg/m², central obesity can be assumed and waist circumference does not need to be measured.
Source: International Diabetes Federation, *The IDF consensus worldwide definition of the Metabolic Syndrome* (2006).

may precipitate awareness of a previously unrecognised diagnosis. An individual may present with an acute myocardial infarction or stroke and be diagnosed with diabetes during his/her first admission to hospital. Alternatively, the patient may very gradually develop symptoms of thirst and polyuria. Established complications, such as retinopathy or albuminuria, may have progressed silently over the preceding years.

Should we screen the population for diabetes?

The early phase of diabetes, in which people are asymptomatic but nevertheless developing serious and preventable complications, would argue strongly in favour of a screening programme. However, while there are numerous identifiable factors that raise an individual's risk, most of them (such as age and body mass index) are very non-specific, so that a screening programme would need to involve a large proportion of the adult population.

A further issue is the choice of screening test. Random blood glucose levels are relatively non-specific, leading to large numbers requiring follow-up, depending on the threshold used. Fasting levels are more specific, but may miss people whose abnormal glucose regulation affects their response to carbohydrate challenge rather than their fasting levels. This is more likely to apply to South Asian people. Such individuals will only be identified by an oral glucose tolerance test (OGTT).

Screening for raised cardiovascular risk

In the UK, the overlap between type 2 diabetes, impaired glucose regulation and raised cardiovascular risk has resulted in a shift away from diabetes screening and towards individualised cardiovascular risk assessments. This is intended for those without either established vascular disease or diabetes in the 40–74 year age group. Such assessments include a random blood glucose estimation, followed by further investigation of borderline or raised levels.

They also involve the use of cardiovascular risk algorithms using the known risk factors, together with other relevant information such as ethnicity, family history, body mass index, waist circumference and random plasma glucose (followed, if necessary, by fasting plasma glucose or OGTT). This serves as a screening programme for vascular risk factors, including diabetes and impaired glucose regulation.

Preventing diabetes in those at risk

Can we delay the onset of diabetes, or prevent it altogether?

The opportunity to reduce cardiovascular risk in individuals with 'pre-diabetes' is one benefit of identifying impaired glucose regulation. Another is the opportunity to delay or prevent progression to diabetes itself. The Diabetes Prevention Programme in the USA (Diabetes Prevention Programme Research Group, 2002) and the Finnish Diabetes Prevention Study (Tuomilehto *et al.*, 2001) both found a 58% reduction in the risk of developing diabetes when such people were treated with lifestyle interventions, including nutritional management, weight loss and exercise (see Figure 4.5 and 4.6). More recently, a study has demonstrated the relationship between adherence to a 'Mediterranean' diet and reduced risk of future diabetes (Martínez-González *et al.*, 2008). The case for drug therapy is more controversial.

Preventing diabetes – lifestyle management or drug therapy?

Drug therapy to prevent diabetes seems an attractive option. While concordance is always an issue, prescribed drug therapy may be adhered to more effectively than lifestyle changes for many individuals. A number of agents have been shown to be effective, summarised in a systematic review by Gillies and colleagues (Gillies *et al.*, 2007). These include metformin, rosiglitazone, acarbose and orlistat. However, a concern is that the drug therapies may be simply masking the onset of diabetes.

There are also practical issues. If we offer a person drug therapy for this reason, at what point do we re-test them for diabetes, and do we withdraw the drug before the test? Unless this policy is very clearly understood, there is a risk that people with impaired glucose regulation may end up with partially treated, undiagnosed diabetes, masked by drug therapy. The diabetes is then not monitored adequately, because the person has never achieved the diagnostic criteria for diabetes and is not on the diabetes register. The importance of the diabetes register as a means of organising diabetes care is emphasised in Chapter 19.

Although trials of behavioural interventions have demonstrated reduced risk of diabetes and cardiovascular disease, there are difficulties in translating these benefits into clinical practice. Even in the more controlled context of a clinical trial involving patients who already have a diagnosis of diabetes, maintaining lifestyle change is not easy. Figure 7.3 in Chapter 7 gives the success rates in the UKPDS study. The Steno-2 study of a multifactorial intervention was similarly affected by fairly low rates of ideal target achievement, particularly for glycaemia and systolic blood pressure (Figure 4.7). Despite this, both studies demonstrated clear benefits for the intervention group.

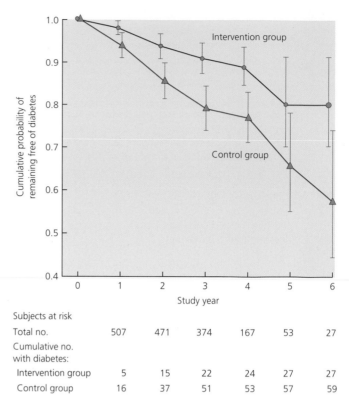

Subjects at risk						
Total no.	507	471	374	167	53	27
Cumulative no. with diabetes:						
Intervention group	5	15	22	24	27	27
Control group	16	37	51	53	57	59

Figure 4.5 Improved risk of developing diabetes in the Finnish Diabetes Prevention Study, which involved a lifestyle intervention. Source: Tuomilehto (2001). Reproduced with permission of *New England Journal of Medicine*.

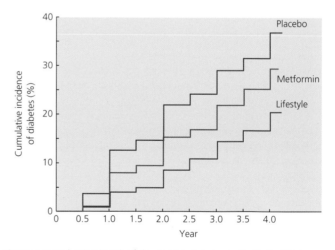

Figure 4.6 Reduction in risk of developing diabetes in the United States Diabetes Prevention Program. The lifestyle intervention reduced the risk by 58% and was significantly more effective than metformin. Source: Tuomilehto (2001). Reproduced with permission of *New England Journal of Medicine*.

The 'missing population' with diabetes

Undiagnosed diabetes in the UK

In addition to those who are known to have diabetes, currently amounting to around 3.5% of the UK population, an estimated 850,000 people have diabetes that is either undiagnosed or

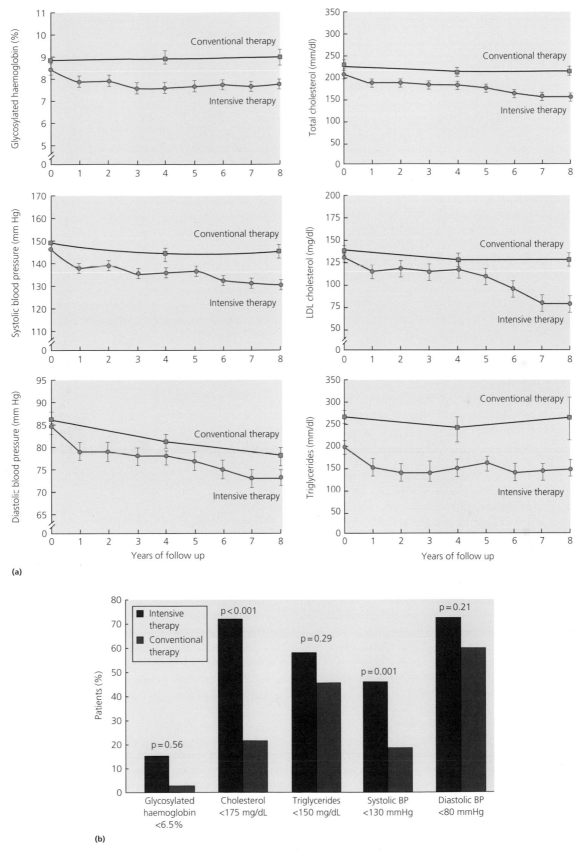

Figure 4.7 Proportion of patients achieving treatment targets in the Steno-2 study. **(a)** Demonstrates significant differences in risk factor levels between the two trial arms. However **(b)** highlights the difficulties in achieving ideal targets, even during a well organised research trial. Source: Gæde *et al.* (2003). Reproduced with permission of *New England Journal of Medicine*.

Box 4.3 **Cornerstones of Early Diabetes Detection**

- Raised awareness of the importance of early detection among the general public and health professionals.
- Low threshold for investigating potential diabetes symptoms.
- Effective follow-up of borderline blood glucose levels (see Box 4.4).
- Active case finding in high-risk groups.
- Regular surveillance in selected patients.

Box 4.4 **Using Primary Care Databases to Identify Undiagnosed Diabetes**

A study published in 2008 Holt *et al.* demonstrated the use of routinely collected general practice data to identify patients at risk of undiagnosed diabetes. The investigators simply looked for raised blood glucose readings in primary care electronic health records. Out of 3.6 million records examined, 0.1% of patients had no diagnosis of diabetes and a random blood glucose level at the most recent measurement ≥ 11.1 mmol/l, or a fasting level ≥ 7.0 mmol/l. This computer search was termed 'Strategy A'.

When projected to the UK population, this would amount to 60,000 individuals. A further 'Strategy B' used a lower threshold of 7.0 mmol/l (random or fasting) for the most recent reading, and identified 0.9% of the survey population, projecting to 528,000 individuals nationwide. Some of these people will have had the reading taken recently and will be in the usual process of follow-up. However, in over a third of the 'A' patients and half of the 'B' patients, the last recorded value was more than one year ago. Some of these people may belong to the missing population with diabetes. As a result of this study, computer software was designed and installed in the majority of UK practices to assist practitioners in identifying them.

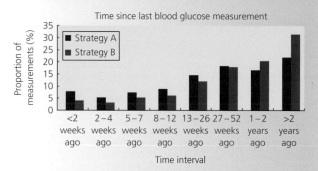

Proportion of blood glucose measurements identified by strategies A and B according to time interval since the measurement.

unrecorded on diabetes registers. These people are failing to receive structured care and follow-up for a serious chronic condition, even in a country with a highly developed health care infrastructure. Adding still further to this problem, large numbers with borderline blood glucose levels are unidentified and likely to suffer highly preventable cardiovascular events. It is this group that are particularly likely to benefit from interventions to prevent diabetes and macrovascular disease.

Raising awareness

Much publicity has been aimed towards the general public to improve early diagnosis of diabetes. This involves two strategies (Box 4.3). Firstly, people should be made aware of the symptoms of diabetes, so that they report them to their health professionals. Secondly, patients in high-risk groups based on ethnicity, family history or other factors should be made aware of arrangements for case finding through regular testing.

Case finding for diabetes

Active measures to detect the 'missing population' with type 2 diabetes include patient awareness raising (e.g. posters encouraging the public to report symptoms of thirst or polyuria), or testing if a family history or other risk factors are present. Health professionals can ensure that people at risk of undiagnosed diabetes are invited for testing (Box 4.4). This includes the following groups:

- Those with features of the metabolic syndrome; see Box 4.1.
- Those with established cardiovascular disease or hypertension, who should have a blood glucose test in some form done every three years. Any random value 6.1 mmol/l or higher should be followed up with a fasting test and HbA1c.
- Those with a family history of type 2 diabetes, particularly in a first-degree relative.
- Ethnic groups, e.g. South Asian, Afro-Caribbean, Hispanic, Pacific Islander.

Investigation of suspicious symptoms

The diagnosis of diabetes is often missed, simply because the condition is not considered as a diagnostic possibility when the individual reports symptoms. Particular settings when this may occur include:

- Failure to include blood glucose or HbA1c measurement in the assessment of tiredness, weight loss or urinary symptoms.
- Investigation of urinary symptoms using a midstream specimen of urine (MSU) that excludes infection, but does not include urinalysis for glucose.

- An assumption that the patient's symptoms are due to prostatic disease, urinary infection, or bladder instability.

This problem often affects type 2 patients, whose symptoms develop gradually and are frequently attributed to ageing. However, an alarming number of type 1 patients are also diagnosed late, and are then at risk of life-threatening ketoacidosis.

Summary

Type 2 diabetes develops gradually and produces non-specific symptoms, so it is often diagnosed late. There is a large missing population with undiagnosed diabetes, and an even larger population with the 'metabolic syndrome', at risk of both diabetes and cardiovascular disease. Opportunities are missed to reduce cardiovascular risk in such patients, whose typically raised body mass index, waist circumference, hypertension and hyperlipidaemia should make them easy to recognise in health care settings. Active programmes of weight reduction, nutritional management and physical activity are proven to reduce progression to diabetes in those at risk, and should be widely promoted. Early detection and intervention are the only means through which the epidemic of diabetes and associated cardiovascular disease can be curtailed. It is among the most important health care challenges of our time.

Further reading and references

Cali AMG, Caprio S (2008). Prediabetes and type 2 diabetes in youth: an emerging epidemic disease? *Current Opinion in Endocrinology, Diabetes & Obesity* **15**, 123–127.

Danaei G, Lawes CMM, Vander Hoorn S *et al.* (2006). Global and regional mortality from ischaemic heart disease and stroke attributable to higher-than-optimum blood glucose concentration: comparative risk assessment. *Lancet* **368**, 1651–1659.

Diabetes Prevention Program Research Group (2002). Reduction in the incidence of type 2 diabetes with lifestyle intervention or metformin. *New England Journal of Medicine* **346**, 393–403.

Gæde P, Vedel P, Larsen N *et al.* (2003). Multifactorial intervention and cardiovascular disease in patients with type 2 diabetes. *New England Journal of Medicine* **348**, 383–393.

Gillies CL, Abrams KR, Lambert PC *et al.* (2007). Pharmacological and lifestyle interventions to prevent or delay type 2 diabetes in people with impaired glucose tolerance: systematic review and meta-analysis. *British Medical Journal* **334**, 299.

Holman R (1998). Assessing the potential for α-glucosidase inhibitors in prediabetic states. *Diabetes Research and Clinical Practice* **40**(Suppl 1), S21-S25.

Holt TA, Stables D, Hippisley-Cox J *et al.* (2008). Identifying undiagnosed diabetes: cross-sectional survey of 3.6 million patients' electronic records. *British Journal of General Practice* **58**, 192–196.

Martínez-González MÁ, de la Fuente-Arrillaga C, Nunez-Cordoba JM (2008). Adherence to Mediterranean diet and risk of developing diabetes: prospective cohort study. *British Medical Journal* **336**, 1348–1351.

Tuomilehto J, Lindström J, Eriksson JG *et al.* (2001). Prevention of type 2 diabetes mellitus by changes in lifestyle among subjects with impaired glucose tolerance. *New England Journal of Medicine* **344**, 1343–1350.

Wild S, Roglic G, Green A *et al.* (2004). Global Prevalence of Diabetes: Estimates for the year 2000 and projections for 2030. *Diabetes Care* **27**, 1047–1053.

CHAPTER 5

Obesity

Tim Holt[1] and Sudhesh Kumar[2]

[1]Nuffield Department of Primary Care Health Sciences, Oxford University, UK
[2]Warwick Medical School, University of Warwick; and WISDEM, University Hospital, Coventry, UK

OVERVIEW

- Obesity is by far the commonest underlying cause of type 2 diabetes today. Even a small amount of weight loss can be beneficial for prevention of type 2 diabetes.

- The clinician must consider active weight management at every stage of type 2 diabetes, as diabetes and associated co-morbidities will also improve with weight loss.

- When treating obesity, the need for good glycaemic control must not be lost sight of. Equally, medication may aggravate obesity, and this must be borne in mind when selecting drugs to treat diabetes and co-morbidities.

- Severe and complex obesity complicated by poor glycaemic control may be treated most effectively by bariatric surgery. In contrast, there is no convincing evidence for effective management of obesity or diabetes and cardiovascular disease through lifestyle changes alone in this group.

Introduction

The global increase in the prevalence of obesity and overweight in the population is fuelling a substantial increase in prevalence of obesity-associated type 2 diabetes. Furthermore, this is also resulting in an early onset of type 2 diabetes, including type 2 diabetes in obese children. Obesity is also increasing the prevalence of special forms of diabetes, such as gestational diabetes. Increasing rates of obesity are also associated with increase in the common co-morbidities with diabetes, such as higher blood pressure and dyslipidaemia. Therefore, obesity management must be considered at virtually every stage of the disease. There are, however, major challenges in that successful behaviour change is essential, and often very difficult to achieve, in those with established severe and complex obesity (obesity with body mass index greater than 35 kg/m²) with diabetes.

Diagnostic criteria

Body Mass Index (BMI), which is calculated using the formula *body weight in kilograms divided by height in metres squared* (mass (kg)/height (m)²), is often used to measure and monitor the degree of obesity. It is, however, an imperfect measurement, as it does not reflect accurately the relationship between body mass and co-morbidities associated with obesity in all ethnic groups or body shapes. Therefore, there is a greater emphasis also on measuring waist circumference, and population-based studies have established 'cut-offs' for abnormal waist circumference in various populations. Waist circumference greater than 94 cm in men and greater than 80 cm indicates central obesity in people of Europid origin.

The use of ethnicity-specific criteria for classification of obesity using BMI has also been recently recognised; for example, South Asian populations have a reduced cut-off at greater than 90 cm for men, but women have the same threshold. Such ethnicity-specific criteria are still not widely implemented, as we have insufficient evidence for the benefit of treatment with drugs, or surgery in particular, at lower levels of BMI in ethnic minority groups. This is an area where further research is needed, but there is no reason why clinical judgement should not be used to make decisions about appropriateness of treatment in ethnic minority groups, where obesity is complicated by poorly controlled diabetes, particularly when recommending lifestyle changes/treatments. The importance of obesity management for prevention of type 2 diabetes is discussed in chapter 11.

Medical management of obesity in diabetic patients

Lifestyle management should be considered the primary modality of treatment and should be considered at all stages of type 2 diabetes. Conceptually, all that is required is a hypo-caloric diet and increase in physical activity to produce sustained reduction in

ABC of Diabetes, Seventh Edition. Tim Holt and Sudhesh Kumar.

Table 5.1 Examples of some classes of prescribed medicines usually associated with weight gain in patients with diabetes.

Anti-diabetic drugs	Insulin
	Sulphonylureas
	Thiazolidinediones
Anti-hypertensive drugs	Beta blockers
Central nervous system drugs	Tricyclic anti-depressants (also used for painful neuropathy)
	Anti-psychotics
	Anti-epileptics

weight. However, the reality is that this requires a fundamental behaviour change in the patient and, while weight loss can be initiated through a variety of diets and exercise interventions, it is usually not sustained, and rebound regain of weight occurs in nearly all patients with diabetes. It is much more difficult to achieve and sustain weight loss in patients with diabetes, even at the early stages of the disease. Furthermore, the number of medications used for management of diabetes and its co-morbidities result in weight gain. Table 5.1 lists some common medications that aggravate weight gain in the obese diabetic patient. Wherever possible, consideration should be given to using alternatives that are weight-neutral instead of these.

Weight loss in obese diabetic patients is associated with improvement in HBA1c. Thus, the degree of improvement in HBA1c is proportional to the degree of weight loss.

Prevention of type 2 diabetes

Some landmark studies have examined the efficacy of obesity management as a strategy for prevention of progression of glucose intolerance to diabetes, and have demonstrated the efficacy of weight reduction. The studies include the US National Institutes of Health (NIH) Diabetes Prevention Programme (DPP) (Knowler *et al.*, 2002) and the Finnish Diabetes Prevention Study (Tuomilehto *et al.*, 2001). A number of other studies have also established the efficacy of this strategy in other populations. However, one difficulty in implementing this approach in usual clinical practice is that it requires significant use of resources, particularly to maintain the behaviour change required. The efficacy of this approach should, however, be borne in mind by the clinician and, wherever possible, every opportunity must be taken to encourage patients to lose weight as soon as impaired glucose intolerance or high risk of diabetes is identified in the obese individual.

Management of obesity through intensive lifestyle modification in patients with diabetes

The efficacy of intensive lifestyle weight management in high-risk patients with existing diabetes was examined recently in the 'Look AHEAD' trial. The hypothesis of this trial was that an intensive weight management programme, producing a weight loss of 7% or more of initial body weight, would reduce the incidence of serious cardiovascular events (cardiovascular death, non-fatal myocardial infarction, hospitalisation with angina, or non-fatal stroke), compared to diabetes support and education. The study was terminated early (after a median follow-up of 9.6 years) because a lack of sufficient efficacy of the intervention at reducing these outcomes was demonstrated, despite mean weight loss of

8.6% of initial body weight (versus 0.7% in controls) in year 1. It may be concluded that lifestyle management alone in type 2 diabetes may not produce reductions in cardiovascular morbidity and mortality on its own. Thus, in such patients, one must not lose sight of the need to control cardiovascular risk factors using drug therapy which is proven to reduce this risk. Furthermore, one must also look beyond lifestyle change alone if sustained weight loss and cardiovascular risk reduction is desirable in the patient.

Drug therapy for obesity

Drug therapy for obesity has had a chequered history because of a large number of failed drugs in the market. This is even more so for patients with type 2 diabetes where, currently, we have a paucity of safe and effective drugs available. There are, however, a number of drugs awaiting a licence for managing obesity in type 2 diabetes, and these may produce additional options for the clinician confronted with an obese individual for whom lifestyle-based therapy alone does not produce the desired weight loss.

There are drugs such as the GLP-1 agonists that, as a class, produce weight loss in a proportion of patients in addition to improvement in diabetes control. These could be considered a preferred option to classes of drugs that aggravate weight gain in those with obesity and type 2 diabetes. The newer SGLT2 inhibitors cause a very modest weight loss, which may also be beneficial in these patients. DPP-4 inhibitors are weight neutral.

Bariatric surgery for patients with diabetes complicated by severe obesity

Bariatric surgery is now becoming increasingly used as a standard of treatment for patients who have poor glycaemic control and have severe and complex obesity. The efficacy of bariatric surgery in such patients is clear and, therefore, it has been recommended by NICE in patients with BMI > 40 kg/m^2 with poorly controlled diabetes, or BMI > 35 kg/m^2 in special cases, including those of some ethnic minorities, such as South Asians with diabetes. The threshold of BMI for which this procedure is recommended is being continually reviewed, as evidence for efficacy becomes available at lower levels. At the present time, however, these are the thresholds for which there is clear evidence of benefits that outweigh the risks.

Organisation of obesity services in a health eco system

Just as diabetes is managed by a number of providers including primary care and specialists, obesity management is also organised along these lines. Obesity management is usually organised in four tiers:

- *Tier 1* is general prevention and public health approaches in an area to reduce weight gain and promote modest weight loss through better lifestyle.
- *Tier 2* is the first level of advice and obesity management, usually carried out in a general practice setting by a 'generalist' – sometimes with professionals such as dieticians. The practice nurse and the general practitioner may choose from a variety of options for lifestyle management and select the option most likely to work for a given patient at a particular time.

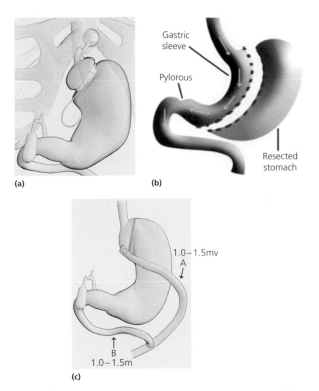

Gastric sleeve

Pylorous

Resected stomach

(a)   (b)

1.0–1.5mv
A
↓

↑
B
1.0–1.5m

(c)

Figure 5.1 Illustrating three common bariatric surgery procedures. **(a)** shows positioning of a gastric band. **(b)** illustrates the sleeve gastrectomy procedure. **(c)** illustrates the gastric bypass procedure. Source: From Vinod Menon, University Hospital Coventry.

Table 5.2 Dietary recommendations pre- and post-operatively.

Pre-op dietary recommendations

Milk and yogurt diet (750–1000 kcal max) – 14 days before surgery:
- Approx 5–8 yoghurts per day depending on calories per pot providing maximum 750 calories per day
- Plus 2 pints or ¾ litre of skimmed/semi skimmed milk per day
- Count the milk you add to tea and coffee
- Sugar free drinks are encouraged throughout the day
- No alcohol

Post-op dietary recommendations

	Gastric band	Sleeve gastrectomy	Gastric bypass
Fluids only	2 weeks	2 weeks	2 weeks
Pureed	2 weeks	2 weeks	2 weeks
Fork-mashable	2 weeks	2 weeks	2 weeks
Solids	Lifelong	Lifelong	Lifelong

Source: From dietetics team at University Hospital Coventry.

b *Sleeve gastrectomy*: Figure 5.1b demonstrates the sleeve gastrectomy operation, which has become more popular in recent years. One sees a significant amount of benefit with respect to weight loss, as with a full gastric bypass, but the operation is considerably less complex and is associated with lower risk. Again, this operation is most commonly done laparoscopically.

c *Full gastric bypass*: there have been several variants of this procedure over the years, and these are now often reserved for patients where behaviour modification is not completely effective. The operation itself produces excellent outcomes for diabetes. However, there is a greater risk of adverse effects with this procedure, as it takes longer than either of the above two procedures. Figure 5.1c illustrates the principles of the procedure.

With these procedures, there is significant benefit in terms of a resolution of diabetes, and an analysis by Buckwald *et al.* (2009) that included a database of 621 studies demonstrated that diabetes was resolved in 75% of patients for more than two years after undergoing bariatric surgery. There are also long-term follow-up studies, such as the Swedish Obesity Study (SOS) (Carlsson *et al.*, 2012), that show the long-term benefits on cardiovascular mortality and morbidity, compared with those patients who do not have surgery and are medically managed.

Post-surgical management of the obese subject with diabetes

It is essential that such patients are managed in a recognised centre that can provide Tier 4 services with a good multidisciplinary team in place. Patients with diabetes with poor control undergoing bariatric surgery require close management by the whole team, including diabetes specialist nurses. During the post-operative period, these patients will require major reductions in anti-diabetic medication and, often, many patients will require no insulin within a day or two of the procedure, especially for procedures like sleeve gastrectomy and gastric bypass. Patients and the clinical teams involved in the surgery may require support from the diabetes specialist teams in managing the reduction of anti-diabetic medication. In a very small number of patients, there is a risk of hypoglycaemia due to nesidioblastosis. This is, however, extremely rare and is the exception.

- When the above fails to produce the required weight loss, it may be necessary to refer patients to a *Tier 3* service, which is a multi-disciplinary service with additional expert input from specialist dieticians, psychologists and, often, an obesity specialist clinician. This may be a specialist in diabetes, but this is not always the case in all localities. What is important is that the multi-disciplinary team work together, as obesity is complex and requires multiple professionals to work together to help achieve the desired outcomes.
- *Tier 4* service is a multi-disciplinary team that is designed for selecting and managing bariatric surgery in patients for whom this is considered the best option.

There are three common approaches to bariatric surgery, namely:

a *Gastric banding*: adjustable gastric bands have become quite popular as the modality of treatment, and Figure 5.1a shows their placement. They work by restricting the passage of food into the stomach and slowing down the consumption of food, such that overall calorie intake is reduced. They do not work in patients who are unable to restrict their carbohydrate intake in particular, and post-operative fallout requires considerable engagement and input from the patient, as adjustments need to made to the band. The patient needs to comply with advice to regulate the intake of certain types of food, to eat more slowly and to eat less overall. Indeed, dietary management and support is essential both pre-operatively and also post-bariatric surgery, and Tables 5.2 describes the approach to common forms of surgery.

Further reading and references

Buchwald H, Estok R, Fahrbach K, Banel D, Jensen MD, Pories WJ, Bantle JP, Sledge I (2009). Weight and type 2 diabetes after bariatric surgery: systematic review and meta-analysis. *American Journal of Medicine* **122**(3), 248–256.

Carlsson LMS, Peltonen M, Ahlin S, *et al.* (2012). Bariatric Surgery and Prevention of Type 2 Diabetes in Swedish Obese Subjects. *New England Journal of Medicine* **367**, 695–704.

Knowler WC, Barrett-Connor E, Fowler SE, Hamman RF, Lachin JM, Walker EA, Nathan DM; Diabetes Prevention Program Research Group (2002). Reduction in the Incidence of Type 2 Diabetes with Lifestyle Intervention or Metformin. *New England Journal of Medicine* **346**, 393–403.

Kushner R, Lawrence V, Kumar S (2013). *Practice Manual of Clinical Obesity.* John Wiley & Sons. ISBN: 978-047065476-7.

NICE Guidelines for Management of Type 2 Diabetes: www.nice.org.uk/cg87

Pories WJ, Swanson MS, McDonald KJ *et al.* (1995). Who would have thought it? An operation proves to be the most effective therapy for adult onset diabetes mellitus. *Annals of Surgery* **222**(3), 339–350

The Look AHEAD Research Group (2013). Cardiovascular Effects of Intensive Lifestyle Intervention in Type 2 Diabetes. *New England Journal of Medicine* **369**, 145–154.

Sjöström L, Narbro K, Sjöström CD *et al.* (2007). Effects of bariatric surgery on mortality in Swedish obese subjects. *New England Journal of Medicine* **357**, 741–752.

Tuomilehto J, Lindström J, Eriksson JG *et al.*; Finnish Diabetes Prevention Study Group (2001). Prevention of type 2 diabetes mellitus by changes in lifestyle among subjects with impaired glucose tolerance. *New England Journal of Medicine* **344**(18), 1343–50.

Wing RR, Koeske R, Epstein LH, Nowalk MP, Gooding W, Becker D (1987). Long-term effects of modest weight-loss in type II diabetic patients. *Archives of Internal Medicine* **147**,1749–1753.

CHAPTER 6

Cardiovascular Disease

Ponnusamy Saravanan[1], Vinod Patel[2], Tim Holt[3] and Sudhesh Kumar[4]

[1]Clinical Sciences Research Institute, Warwick Medical School, Coventry; and George Eliot Hospital, Nuneaton, UK
[2]Institute of Clinical Education, Warwick Medical School, Coventry; and George Eliot Hospital, Nuneaton, UK
[3]Nuffield Department of Primary Care Health Sciences, Oxford University, UK
[4]Warwick Medical School, University of Warwick; and WISDEM, University Hospital, Coventry, UK

OVERVIEW

- Macrovascular disease, including myocardial infarction and stroke, is the prime cause of excess mortality in diabetes.

- Microvascular disease produces disabling complications, including retinopathy and nephropathy.

- Vascular outcomes are improved through multifactorial interventions.

- Tight control of glycaemia, blood pressure and serum cholesterol usually requires a combination of lifestyle change and several different drug therapies.

- Angiotensin-converting enzyme inhibitors are the drugs of first choice for hypertension in people with diabetes, unless they are of Afro-Caribbean descent, or where there is a possibility of pregnancy.

Introduction

Most people with type 2 diabetes will ultimately die from cardiovascular disease – and many of these, prematurely. People with type 2 diabetes have a doubled risk of CVD, even after adjustment for the well-established risk factors (Seshasai *et al.*, 2011). Vascular complications are highly preventable, provided good quality, target-driven care is maintained consistently throughout the individual's life.

Life expectancy is reduced in people with diabetes (Figures 6.1–6.3) for a number of reasons; preventable cardiovascular disease remains the major one. Effective control of cardiovascular risk requires a multifactorial approach, as described in this chapter (Box 6.1).

'Buying in' to polypharmacy

In many areas of medicine, polypharmacy is rightly seen in a negative light. With increasing drugs in the regimen, interactions become more common. Patient adherence may be problematical, particularly on divided dose regimens, with the risk of accidental overdosing. Reactions to medication may occur that are difficult to attribute to a single component of the schedule. All of these problems are more common in the elderly and, particularly, in the visually impaired, who may need supervision from a carer and dosette boxes or other aids.

However, in diabetes, a multifactorial approach will inevitably require multiple drug therapies. This is not always particularly acceptable to patients, who sometimes feel that the risks of polypharmacy cannot possibly be outweighed. So how do we manage expectations and facilitate the introduction of what is likely for most patients to be a regimen of at least three different drugs?

Explain *at the outset* why polypharmacy in diabetes is worth the potential difficulties. Mention the probable need for multiple therapies to prevent CVD – particularly strokes and heart disease – in the first place. The addition of a second or third antihypertensive may then be accepted as a norm and not seen as a simple 'failure' of monotherapy. It is very important to communicate the evidence for this approach directly to patients. For example, statins such as atorvastatin 10 mg reduced strokes by 48% and acute coronary events by 36% in the CARDS study (Box 6.2).

The commonly used drugs are safe for the majority. Controlling blood pressure using two or more different agents is more likely to be successful than using higher doses of single drugs, and less likely to give the side-effects that are often associated with the higher- rather than middle-range doses. The same principle applies to other areas, including glycaemic control where, for instance, metformin may be increased from a moderate dose to the maximum licensed dose with little improvement in blood glucose levels but significantly greater risk of abdominal side effects. With respect to metformin, it is important to note that the slow-release formulation is usually much better tolerated. For hypertension, effective control may be achieved if more than one pathway is blocked, preventing the system from escaping the effects of a single-pathway approach. Explaining these principles to the patient may begin to put the concept of polypharmacy in a more positive light.

ABC of Diabetes, Seventh Edition. Tim Holt and Sudhesh Kumar.

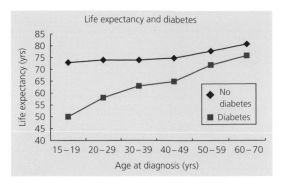

Figure 6.1 Life expectancy is reduced in diabetes, particularly for the young type 1 patients diagnosed in childhood. This figure is based on a mortality study reported in the 1970s. Modern proactive prevention programmes with tight risk factor control and early intervention for emerging complications are changing this pattern. Source: Goodkin (1975). Reproduced with permisison of Wolters Kluwer Health.

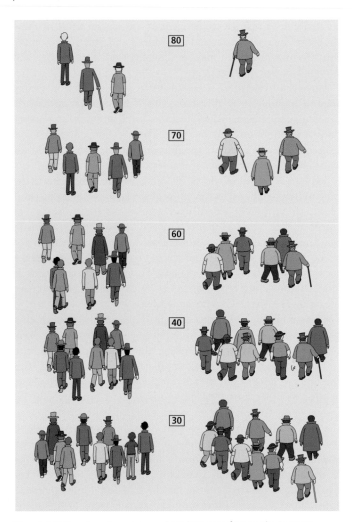

Figure 6.2 How ten obese men and ten lean men fare on the journey through life. Source: Joslin (1941).

Blood glucose control

Blood glucose control is particularly important for the prevention of microvascular complications, including retinopathy, nephropathy, and peripheral and autonomic neuropathies. Table 6.1 shows the impact found in a number of studies.

Glycaemic control has a less substantial, but still important, impact on macrovascular disease (Figure 6.4). The intensive treatment group in the UKPDS study showed 16% fewer myocardial infarctions (Figure 6.5). This study also demonstrated that metformin therapy provided additional CVD benefit over and above the glucose-lowering effect, and should therefore be initiated in all type 2 patients, along with the lifestyle advice. The UKPDS metformin study cohort was relatively small in comparison with more recent studies in diabetes, with only 342 allocated metformin versus 411 on diet and other glucose-lowering treatments. The 39% relative risk reduction in MI and 36% reduction in all-cause mortality justifies the early use of metformin in diabetes care. There is also emerging evidence that metformin improves glycaemic control by approximately 0.6 HbA1c%, and can be insulin-sparing in patients with type 1 diabetes. In the STOP-NIDDM trial of patients with impaired glucose tolerance, acarbose significantly reduced the number of CVD events, suggesting that control of post-prandial hyperglycaemia may be beneficial. However, this needs to be proved in prospective studies.

Initial management of blood glucose depends largely on the type of diabetes and the presenting clinical picture. A specific guide is provided in Chapter 7 for type 2 patients.

Tight glycaemic control in older patients – balancing risks and benefits

Increasing numbers of type 2 patients are commencing insulin in order to achieve tight glycaemic control. The benefits of reduced HbA1c need to be balanced against the disadvantages, including the risk of hypoglycaemia. Severe hypoglycaemia may require hospital admission and has a detrimental impact on quality of life.

The intensive glucose-lowering arm of the ACCORD study had to be halted, due to an excess of deaths in those aiming for HbA1c of 42 mmol/mol or less, although the cause of these deaths was not simply hypoglycaemia. These findings have triggered a debate about the priority given to tight, rather than simply adequate, glycaemic control in type 2 diabetes, where it could be argued that the major issue is macrovascular disease, unless microvascular complications are established.

Blood pressure control

Antihypertensive medication will be required in the majority of type 2 patients to achieve a target of < 140/80 mm Hg. This should be complemented with lifestyle advice to increase exercise and reduce weight and salt and alcohol consumption, if appropriate.

Choice of initial antihypertensive therapy

Patients with diabetes whose blood pressure is not within the 140/80 target should be offered antihypertensive drug therapy. First line choice should be an angiotensin-converting enzyme (ACE) inhibitor, unless the person is of Afro-Caribbean descent, or if there is a possibility of pregnancy. In such cases, a calcium channel blocker is appropriate. If the target is still not achieved, a calcium channel blocker or diuretic should then be offered. All three drugs may be given if successful control is still not achieved. The Micro-HOPE study results showed that Ramipril 10 mg reduces the composite outcome of MI, stroke or CV death by 34%. (Heart Outcomes Prevention Evaluation Study Investigators, 2000).

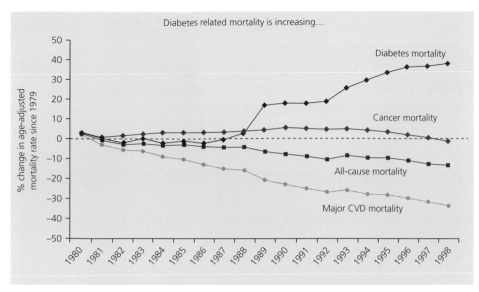

Figure 6.3 Although overall cardiovascular mortality is declining, its rate in the population with diabetes is increasing (based on US data). Source: Sobel *et al.* (2003). Reproduced with permission of American Heart Association.

Box 6.1 **Microvascular and Macrovascular Disease**

Tight glycaemic control is particularly effective at reducing microvascular complications (retinopathy, nephropathy, neuropathy), while macrovascular disease affecting the larger vessels is more influenced by lipids, blood pressure, body fat distribution and exercise. Blood pressure control (and smoking cessation) has a highly beneficial effect on both micro- and macrovascular disease. Therefore, a multifactorial approach, addressing all of these factors, is extremely important.

Box 6.2 **The CARDS Study**

The CARDS Study demonstrated a reduction of major cardiovascular events of 37% in people with type 2 diabetes with normal LDL cholesterol levels, treated with 10 mg of atorvastatin (see Tables 6.2 and 6.3). Stroke risk was reduced by 48%, and the treatment effect was independent of the pre-treatment cholesterol value. It would appear that patients with diabetes benefit even if their total cholesterol is less than 4 mmol/l.

Table 6.1 Reductions in HbA1c and corresponding reductions in microvascular and macrovascular complications described in major studies of people with type 1 and type 2 diabetes.

Study name	DCCT	UKPDS	Kumamoto	Steno-2
HbA1c	↓2%	↓0.9%	↓2%	↓1.0%
Retinopathy	↓63%	↓17–21%	↓69%	↓58%
Nephropathy	↓54%	↓24–33%	↓70%	↓61%
Autonomic neuropathy	↓60%	–	–	↓63%
CVD	↓41%	↓16%	–	↓53%

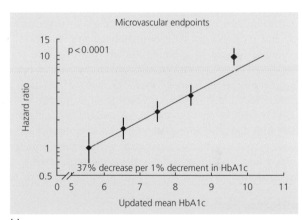

(a)

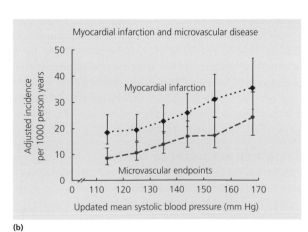

(b)

Figure 6.4 (a) Glycaemic control improves microvascular outcomes. **(b)** Blood pressure control reduces risk of both macro- and microvascular complications. Source: Stratton *et al.*, (2000). Reproduced with permission of BMJ Publishing Group.

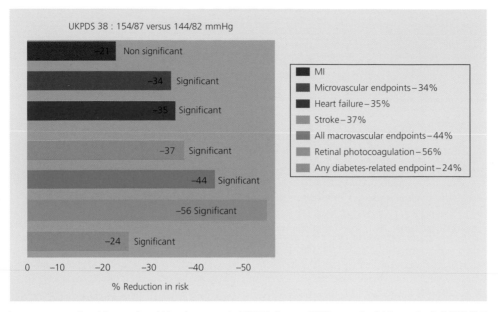

UKPDS 38 : 154/87 versus 144/82 mmHg

-21 Non significant
-34 Significant
-35 Significant
-37 Significant
-44 Significant
-56 Significant
-24 Significant

■ MI
■ Microvascular endpoints – 34%
■ Heart failure – 35%
■ Stroke – 37%
■ All macrovascular endpoints – 44%
■ Retinal photocoagulation – 56%
■ Any diabetes-related endpoint – 24%

0   -10   -20   -30   -40   -50
% Reduction in risk

Figure 6.5 Reductions in outcomes attributable to reduced blood pressure in UKPDS. Source: UK Prospective Diabetes Study (UKPDS) Group (1998). Reproduced with permission of BMJ Publishing Group.

Renal impairment and albuminuria

Microalbuminuria and proteinuria

A positive finding of microalbumin should be confirmed on a second sample and, if this is negative, a third sample should be checked. An MSU should be sent to exclude infection. Once confirmed, the patient should be treated with an ACE inhibitor or ARBs (angiotensin receptor blocker)) if tolerated, even if their blood pressure is normal, and tighter targets for blood pressure (130/80 mm Hg or lower) and HbA1c (aim for 6.5%) should be set, tailored to the individual. Patients with diabetes and hypertension who have dipstick-positive *proteinuria* (not just microalbuminuria) usually have widespread vascular disease, and are at high risk of cardiovascular events. All of these patients should also be treated with an ACE inhibitor or ARB.

Monitoring renal function

Patients with diabetes are at higher risk of renal impairment – particularly older patients who also have hypertension, or those with any degree of proteinuria or microalbuminuria. All patients with diabetes should have estimated glomerular filtration rate (e-GFR) measured at least annually, and many will require more frequent testing. Estimated GFR is a more satisfactory marker of renal function than creatinine alone. Patients with established diabetic nephropathy will require further assessment through 24-hour urinary protein excretion and measurement of actual (rather than estimated) GFR (see also Chapter 13).

Starting ACE inhibitors or A2RBs

All patients treated with an ACE inhibitor or ARB should have their potassium and creatinine checked prior to starting these agents, and again after 7–10 days, to ensure that hyperkalaemia or increased creatinine has not occurred. This should be repeated at every dose change. A 10–15% increase in creatinine is tolerated by most renal physicians, but seek local advice. Estimated GFR is a more adequate measure of renal function than creatinine alone in this situation.

Lipid lowering in people with diabetes

Most people with diabetes, particularly those over 40 years, should be considered at risk of cardiovascular disease (Box 6.2). Some are at higher risk than others, and lower risk-type 2 patients should have their risk reassessed annually (see Box 6.3).

If the person is considered not to be at high cardiovascular risk, estimate cardiovascular risk annually using the QRISK2 equation. If the risk of a cardiovascular event is 10% or higher, lipid modification using drug therapy (atorvastatin 20 mg daily) should be offered (Table 6.2), in addition to a cardioprotective diet (see Chapter 12).

Targets

Recommended targets for cholesterol lowering in diabetes are:
- Total cholesterol < **4.0** mmol/l
- LDL < **2.0** mmol/l

Note that LDL can only be measured accurately on a fasting sample (like triglycerides) but, for most monitoring purposes, random total cholesterols are adequate once control is achieved. In people with no history of cardiovascular events, the currently recommended treatment in the UK is to use atorvastatin 20 mg daily. Those with such a history are treated with atorvastatin 80 mg daily.

Choice of drug

The best quality RCT evidence in diabetes care in relation to lipid-lowering is the CARDS study (Table 6.3). The statin used in that study was atorvastatin 10 mg daily. Atorvastatin is generally better tolerated than simvastatin, and has fewer clinically important drug interactions. For example, simvastatin is contraindicated with ciclosporin or danazol or gemfibrozil. More importantly, the recommended maximum dose of simvastatin is 40 mg, and with amlodipine or diltiazem it is only 20 mg. Atorvastatin is well tolerated at higher doses (40 mg or 80 mg).

On commencing statins, patients should be advised to report unexplained myalgia or muscle weakness. Statin-induced myositis

Box 6.3 **NICE Recommendation for Cardiovascular Risk Assessment:**

Consider a person to be at high premature cardiovascular risk for his or her age, unless he or she:

- is not overweight, tailoring this with an assessment of body weight associated risk according to ethnic group
- is normotensive (<140/80 mmHg in the absence of antihypertensive therapy)
- does not have microalbuminuria
- does not smoke
- does not have a high-risk lipid profile
- has no history of cardiovascular disease, and
- has no family history of cardiovascular disease

Table 6.2 CHD prevention trials with statins in diabetes.

Study	Drug	Number of patients	CHD risk reduction non-diabetics	CHD risk reduction diabetes
Primary prevention				
CARDS	Atorvastatin 10 mg	2838		37%*
HPS[†]	Simvastatin 40 mg	2912	25%[‡]	26–33%
Secondary prevention				
CARE[§]	Pravastatin	586	23%	
4S[¶]	Simvastatin	202	32%	55%
GREACE	Atorvastatin 24 mg	313		59%
4S reanalysis**	Simvastatin	483	32%	42%
HPS	Simvastatin	3051	24%[‡]	12% NS

CHD endpoints:
* CARDS, acute coronary events
[†] HPS, first major vascular event
[§] CARE, absolute risk of coronary events
[¶] 4S major CHD events
** 4S reanalysis, major coronary events.
Cohorts:
[‡] HPS, risk reduction for the entire cohort (non-diabetics and patients with diabetes).
NS, not statistically significant.

Table 6.3 Cardiovascular disease outcomes in the CARDS study.

	Placebo (n = 1410)	Atorvastatin (n = 1428)
Type of first event		
Fatal myocardial infarction	20	8
Other acute coronary heart disease death	4	10
Non-fatal myocardial infarction*	41	25
Unstable angina	9	7
Resuscitated cardiac arrest	0	0
Coronary revascularisation	18	12
Fatal stroke	5	1
Non-fatal stroke	30	20
Total	127	83

*Five silent myocardial infarctions included in each group.

is not common, but it can be a serious problem if the drug is not withdrawn. However, mild muscle aches without evidence of myositis are much commoner, and are not necessarily an indication for statin withdrawal.

Fibrates are appropriate drugs for those intolerant of statins, but they can also cause myopathy. They can also be used as second line in those not achieving control with statins alone, or if fasting triglycerides remain raised above 2.3 mmol/l despite statin therapy. Fenofibrate has good evidence for reduction in some diabetes complications (FIELD Study), and has far fewer interactions than gemfibrozil. In patients with previous myocardial infarction, omega-3 fatty acids have been shown to reduce CVD and all-cause mortality. They may also be used if hypertriglyceridaemia persists despite fibrate therapy.

Other ways of reducing cardiovascular risk

Smoking cessation

In a person with diabetes, smoking is particularly harmful. It not only increases the already raised risk of macrovascular disease, but also increases microvascular complications, particularly nephropathy and retinopathy. Patients with diabetes who smoke should be actively targeted for smoking cessation interventions.

Use of low dose aspirin

Recent trials suggest that, despite their raised cardiovascular risk, people with diabetes may not, in fact, benefit from low dose aspirin as previous guidelines advised, and further research is needed to clarify this issue. However a meta-analysis and review from the ADA suggests the following with respect to low-dose aspirin (75 mg daily) for primary prevention of CVD. This takes into account the fact people with diabetes are not a homogeneous group with respect to their CVD risk.

- **High risk group**: Low-dose aspirin is recommended for primary CVD prevention in adults with diabetes who are at increased CVD risk (ten-year risk of CVD events over 10%), and who are not at increased risk for bleeding (e.g. peptic ulcer disease, warfarin, regular NSAID use). This group will include most men over age 50 years, and women over age 60 years who have one or more of the following risk factors: smoking, hypertension, dyslipidemia, family history of premature CVD, micro-albuminuria, proteinuria.
- **Intermediate risk group**: Low-dose aspirin use for prevention might be considered for those with diabetes at intermediate CVD risk (younger patients with one or more risk factors, or older patients with no risk factors, or patients with ten-year CVD risk of 5–10%) according to patient choice and clinician discretion.
- **Low risk group**: Aspirin should not be recommended for primary CVD prevention at low CVD risk (men under age 50 years and women under 60 years with no major additional CVD risk factors; ten-year CVD risk under 5%), as the potential adverse effects from bleeding offset the potential benefits.

Anti-obesity drugs

There is increasing interest in the pharmacological treatment of obesity, but this approach should be part of a structured programme of monitoring and follow-up if it is to be effective. Any management of obesity should have a primary focus on optimizing weight, via an individualised plan based on sufficient physical activity, dietary review with some calorie restriction, and promoting healthy eating behaviours, including safe alcohol consumption.

Licensed preparations available in the UK include orlistat only. Obesity drugs are discussed further in Chapter 5.

Physical activity and exercise

Physical activity and exercise are important means of reducing cardiovascular risk as part of a multifactorial package of interventions (see below). Without regular exercise, attempts to lose weight are much less likely to succeed. Any amount of physical activity is beneficial, but a regular habit of moderate physical activity for at least 30 minutes on five days of the week is recommended for all patients if at all possible, as it is for the general public.

People with diabetes should be specifically advised that moderate-intensity activity should be enough to raise the heart rate, resulting in breathing faster and feeling warmer. A good indicator is that the person should still be able to talk, but not sing a song!

Muscle-strengthening activities on two or more days a week that work all major muscle groups (legs, hips, back, abdomen, chest, shoulders and arms) are also recommended by the NHS. Examples of muscle-strengthening activities include:

- lifting weights;
- working with resistance bands;
- doing exercises that use your body weight for resistance, such as push-ups and sit-ups;
- heavy gardening, such as digging and shovelling;
- yoga.

Multifactorial interventions in diabetes care

Most existing trial evidence is based on the effect of a single intervention on CVD outcomes. Very few well-designed studies on multifactorial interventions have been published to date. A seminal study in this regard was Steno-2, which provided evidence of the cardiovascular benefits of multifactorial intervention in diabetes (Figure 6.6). 160 type 2 patients with microalbuminuria were randomised to receive conventional treatment in accordance to national Danish guidelines, or to an intensive treatment arm. This involved stepwise implementation of behaviour modification and pharmacological treatment that targeted hyperglycaemia, hypertension, dyslipidaemia, microalbuminuria and secondary prevention of cardiovascular disease with aspirin. At the end of the 7.8 year study period, there were significant reductions in HbA1c%, systolic and diastolic blood pressure, serum cholesterol and triglycerides, and urine albumin excretion in the treatment group. Patients receiving intensive treatment had a significantly lower risk of cardiovascular disease by about 50%.

At the end of the treatment period, all the patients were offered intensive treatment and were further followed up for an additional 6.5 years. Despite convergence of most of the risk factors between the groups, there was an additional benefit in CVD events in the original intensive treatment group. This suggests that treatment

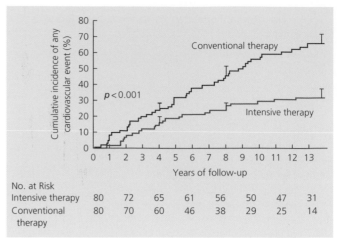

(a)

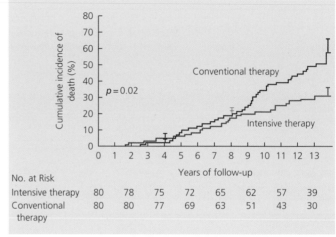

(b)

Figure 6.6 Cumulative incidence of cardiovascular events **(a)**, and of death **(b)** in the Steno-2 study. Source: Gaede *et al.* (2003). Reproduced with permission of *The New England Journal of Medicine*.

of multiple risk factors should be started early. The specific reductions, comparing the previously intensive group to the conventional group, were as follows:

- All deaths by 46%.
- CVD death by 57%.
- Cardiovascular events by 59%.
- Laser treatment for diabetic retinopathy by 55%.
- End-stage renal failure, one patient versus six patients.

There is other trial evidence for multi-factorial intervention. Figure 6.7 shows a little-known depiction of the effects of BP and glycaemic control from the UKPDS study. It clearly shows that, to minimize diabetes complications, both the BP and glycaemic control need to be targeted in all patients with diabetes. In the ASCOT study, there was clear evidence of synergy between a BP-lowering strategy based on amlodipine/perindopril and lipid-lowering with atorvastatin. A considerable number of patients with diabetes were enrolled in this study, and the authors concluded that there was a 79% reduction in actual CHD events compared with that

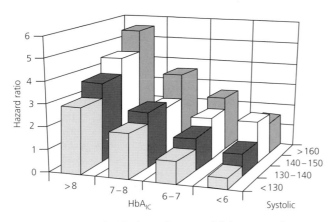

Figure 6.7 UKPDS Study risk of complications of diabetes according to BP and glycaemic control quartiles. Source: Mogensen (2000). Reproduced with permission of BMJ.

Box 6.4 **The Alphabet Strategy**

An ideal management programme should, as a minimum, address the following issues in the Alphabet Strategy format:

Advice: Education, self-management, compliance. Special focus on optimising physical activity, diet, weight reduction, cessation of smoking.

Blood pressure: Optimal control usually less than 130/80 mm Hg; in most cases initial treatment will be with an ACE inhibitor/ARB, often in combination with a thiazide-like diuretic.

Cholesterol treatment: Target total cholesterol < 4.0 mmol/l, LDL < 2.0 mmol/l, HDL > 1.0 mmol/l and triglycerides < 1.7 mmol/l. Statins in most cases.

Diabetes control: Ideal HbA1c target 6.5% (48 mmol/mol). Individualise to patient. Metformin first line in most patients. Early recourse to multiple therapy and insulin if targets not reached.

Eye care: Detailed yearly examination and appropriate referral. Aggressive management of vascular risk factors if retinopathy is present.

Feet care: Detailed yearly examination and appropriate referral. Aggressive management of vascular risk factors if neuropathy and peripheral vascular disease is present.

Guardian drugs: Microalbuminuria/proteinuria patients should be considered for ACE inhibitors or ARB. Statins for secondary prevention and primary prevention.

Alphabet Strategy Care Plans are available to download from www. abcdiabetescare.org.uk

expected from the Framingham risk calculation for the cohort (Sever *et al.*, 2009).

The Alphabet Strategy is an 'ABC of reducing diabetes complications' published in 2002 and is summarised in Boxes 6.4 and 6.5. Evidence indicates that it can help deliver the same targets that were achieved in trials of multi-factorial intervention, specifically UKPDS and Steno-2 (Javieer *et al.*, 2003; see Table 6.4).

Box 6.5 **Alphabet Strategy Advice for Patients**

1 Do not smoke.
2 Maintain ideal body weight for adults (body mass index 20–25 kg/m²) and avoid central obesity (waist circumference in white Caucasians < 102 cm in men and < 88 cm in women, and in Asians < 90 cm in men and < 80 cm in women.
3 Keep total dietary intake of fat to ≤ 30% of total energy intake.
4 Keep intake of saturated fats to ≤ 10% of total fat intake.
5 Keep intake of dietary cholesterol to < 300 mg/day.
6 Replace saturated fats by an increased intake of monounsaturated fats.
7 Increase intake of fresh fruit and vegetables to at least five portions per day.
8 Regular intake of fish and other sources of omega-3 fatty acids (at least two servings of fish per week).
9 Limit alcohol intake to < 21 units/week for men or < 14 units/week for women.
10 Limit intake of salt to < 100 mmol/l day (<6 g of sodium chloride or < 2.4 g of sodium per day).
11 Regular aerobic physical activity of at least 30 minutes per day, most days of the week, should be taken (for example, fast walking/swimming).

Table 6.4 Summary of targets achieved in the Steno-2 Study adapted to the Alphabet Strategy.

	Intensive treatment cohort	Conventional treatment cohort
Advice	Standard	
Blood pressure	131/73	146/78
Cholesterol	TC: 3.5 mmol/l	TC: 5mmol/l
	LDL: 1.8 mmol/l	
Diabetes control	7.9%	9%
Eyes	Annual check	Annual check
Feet	Annual check	Annual check
Guardian drugs	85% on statin, ACE-1 or ARB	<50% on statin, ACE-1 or ARB

Source: Data from STENO Study.

Summary

The main focus of diabetes care should revolve around improving the life of the individual through reducing the impact of diabetes. This will be by using simple treatment regimes that have minimal interference with daily living. The treatment regimes must be based on good quality clinical evidence, and should be affordable to the society in which they are implemented. There is accumulating evidence to suggest that multi-factorial intervention is key to reducing almost all the complications of diabetes, such as CVD, retinopathy, nephropathy, lower limb amputation and neuropathy.

Modifiable risk factors include blood pressure, blood glucose, lipids, obesity, low physical activity, smoking and albuminuria. Management of these risk factors involves a combination of lifestyle and pharmacological approaches, tailored to individual patient preferences.

Further reading and references

Action to Control Cardiovascular Risk in Diabetes (ACCORD) Study Group (2008). Effects of Intensive Glucose Lowering in Type 2 Diabetes. *New England Journal of Medicine* **358**(24), 2545–2559.

Colhoun HM, Betteridge DJ, Durrington PN *et al.* (2004). Primary prevention of cardiovascular disease with atorvastatin in type 2 diabetes in the Collaborative Atorvastatin Diabetes Study (CARDS): multicentre randomised placebo-controlled trial. *Lancet* **364**, 685–696.

Gaede P, Vedel P, Larsen N (2003). Multifactorial intervention and cardiovascular disease in patients with type 2 diabetes. *New England Journal of Medicine* **348**, 383–93.

Goodkin G (1975). Mortality factors in diabetes. A 20 year mortality study. *Journal of Occupational Medicine* **17**(11), 716–721.

Heart Outcomes Prevention Evaluation Study Investigators (2000). Effects of Ramipril on cardiovascular and microvascular outcomes in people with type 2 diabetes: results of the HOPE and MICRO-HOPE substudy. *Lancet* **355**, 253–9.

Javieer P, Saraswathy J, Lee J, Morrissey J, Patel V (2003). The alphabet strategy – A tool to achieve clinical trial standards in routine practice? *British Journal Of Diabetes And Vascular Disease* **3**, 410–413.

Mogensen CM (2000). Diabetic nephropathy: evidence for renoprotection and practice. *Heart* **84**(Suppl I), i26–i28.

National Institute of Health and Clinical Excellence (2008). *Diabetes-type 2 (update) CG66.*

Ohkubo Y, Kishikawa H, Araki E, Miyata T, Isami S, Motoyoshi S *et al.* (1995). Intensive insulin therapy prevents the progression of diabetic microvascular complications in Japanese patients with non-insulin-dependent diabetes mellitus: a randomized prospective 6 year study. *Diabetes Research and Clinical Practice* **28**, 103–117.

Patel V, Morrissey J (2002). The Alphabet Strategy: The ABC of reducing diabetes complications. *British Journal of Diabetes and Vascular Disease* **2**, 58–59.

Pignone M, Alberts MJ, Colwell JA *et al.* (2010). Aspirin for Primary Prevention of Cardiovascular Events in People With Diabetes. A position statement of the American Diabetes Association. *Diabetes Care* **33**(6), 1395–1402.

Seshasai SR, Kaptoge S, Thompson A *et al.* and the Emerging Risk Factors Collaboration (2011). Diabetes Mellitus, fasting glucose, and risk of cause-specific death. *New England Journal of Medicine* **364**, 829–841.

Sever PS, Poulter NR, Lan Chang C, Dahlof B, Wedel H, on behalf of the ASCOT Investigators (2009). Coronary heart disease benefits from blood pressure and lipid-lowering. *International Journal of Cardiology* **135**, 218–222.

Sobel BE, Frye R, Detre KM *et al.* (2003). Burgeoning dilemmas in the management of diabetes and cardiovascular disease: rationale for the Bypass Angioplasty Revascularization Investigation 2 Diabetes (BARI 2D) Trial. *Circulation* **107**, 636–642.

Stevens RJ, Kothari V, Adler AI *et al.* on behalf of the United Kingdom Prospective Diabetes Study (UKPDS) Group (2001). The UKPDS risk engine: a model for the risk of coronary heart disease in Type II diabetes (UKPDS 56). *Clinical Science* **101**, 671–679.

Stratton IM, Adler AI, Neil HA *et al.* (2000). Association of glycaemia with macrovascular and microvascular complications of type 2 diabetes (UKPDS 35): prospective observational study. *BMJ* **321**(7258), 405–412.

UK Prospective Diabetes Study (UKPDS) Group (1998a). Intensive blood-glucose control with sulphonylureas or insulin compared with conventional treatment and risk of complications in patients with type 2 diabetes (UKPDS 33). *Lancet* **352**, 837–853.

UK Prospective Diabetes Study (UKPDS) Group (1998b). Effect of intensive blood-glucose control with metformin on complications in overweight patients with type 2 diabetes (UKPDS 34). *Lancet* **352**, 854–865.

CHAPTER 7

Management of Blood Glucose in Type 2 Diabetes

Tim Holt[1] and Sudhesh Kumar[2]

[1]Nuffield Department of Primary Care Health Sciences, Oxford University, UK
[2]Warwick Medical School, University of Warwick; and WISDEM, University Hospital, Coventry, UK

OVERVIEW

- Structured education, life-style change, and drug therapy are keys to successful glycaemic control in type 2 diabetes.

- The majority can be managed in primary care, using an expanding range of therapeutic options.

- An increasing proportion of patients require insulin to achieve target HbA1c.

- Patients should be reviewed every 2–3 months until their personal glycaemic target is achieved, and six-monthly thereafter.

Introduction

The rising prevalence of type 2 diabetes and increasing recognition of undiagnosed patients means that each general practice will be regularly making new diagnoses. Most of these patients will not be acutely unwell, and some will be asymptomatic and detected on biochemical tests. Modern management of type 2 diabetes involves early effective control of hyperglycaemia through patient education and drug therapy, including insulin if needed. The majority of this can be carried out in primary care, given sufficient practice-based expertise and, where necessary, access to secondary care resources.

While there is evidence of safety and efficacy for individual drugs, there is less evidence available on which particular treatment algorithm is most effective for the management of type 2 diabetes. Guidelines are, therefore, based on expert consensus reports, rather than robust evidence. Although the broad principles are similar, there may be significant differences between different guidelines issued by various professional bodies.

Initial management

If a patient has been diagnosed early, with no symptoms or complications and an HbA1c < 53 mmol/mol at diagnosis, and if they prefer a time without drug therapy, then an initial three months of behavioural adaptation is appropriate. However, a patient with symptoms or a raised HbA1c at diagnosis has probably had diabetes for some time already, and there is then a good case for starting metformin immediately to improve control. There is increasing recognition of the benefits of early blood glucose control on long-term outcomes, a phenomenon that has been termed 'glycaemic memory'.

Lifestyle advice

This is important throughout the course of diabetes and not just at the start. It should be reinforced at each review, even though further drug therapy may be added. Dietary advice and advice on exercise is part of structured education, as discussed in Chapter 3.

Monitoring HbA1c

HbA1c should be checked every three months, with action taken each time until the level is at, or moving towards, the patient-specific target, and then every six months after the target has been achieved.

Drug therapy options

There is now a wide range of treatment options for lowering blood glucose in type 2 diabetes (see Figure 7.1).

Key issues in selecting the best option are:

- Metformin is recommended first line for most type 2 patients.
- Sulphonylureas have a more immediate effect at reducing blood glucose levels in symptomatic patients, and may also be first choice for insulin-deficient individuals.
- Sulphonylureas, glitazones and insulin may all cause weight gain, and obesity is often already a problem.
- Sulphonylureas may put the patient at risk of hypoglycaemia, with implications for driving.
- There appears to be increased risk of distal fractures in women using pioglitazone.
- Pioglitazone may cause fluid retention, exacerbating or precipitating heart failure, and may be associated with an increased risk of bladder cancer.

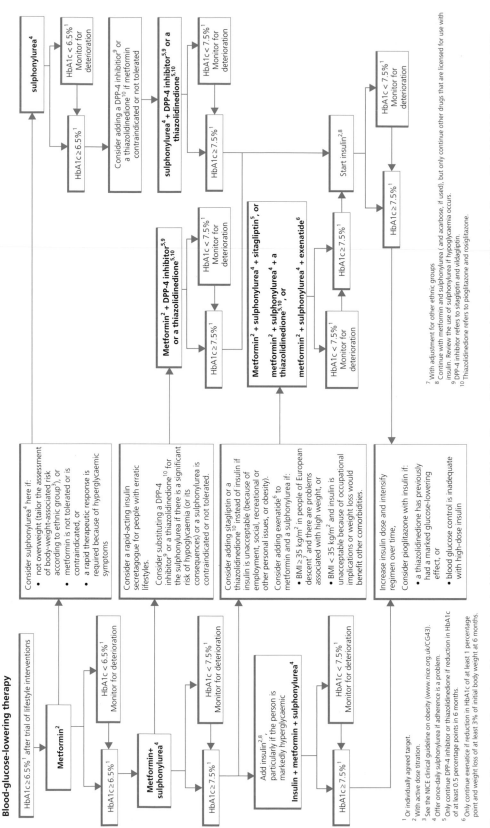

Figure 7.1 Treatment pathway to guide management of blood glucose in type 2 diabetes. Source: National Institute for Health and Clinical Excellence, Clinical Guideline 87 (2009). NICE guidelines are revised periodically and readers should check the most recent publication. Reproduced with permission of NICE.

- GLP-1 analogues (Exenatide, Liraglutide, Lixisenatide) may assist with weight reduction.
- The 'gliptins' are weight-neutral and do not raise the risk of hypoglycaemia unless added in with a sulphonylurea or glinide.
- No dose adjustment is required for Linagliptin in patients with renal impairment.
- Failure of the HbA1c to respond to GLP-1 or a gliptin after an appropriate interval requires withdrawal of the drug.

First line

The majority of patients, and certainly those who are overweight (BMI $\geq$ 25 kg/m^{-2}), should start metformin first line. This should be started at 500 mg once or twice a day, and the dose increased after 5–7 days (see Box 7.1). Increasing the dose gradually may offset the gastrointestinal side effects that many patients fail to tolerate (Box 7.2).

Non-obese patients may be insulin-deficient (particularly if they have actually lost weight) and could start a sulphonylurea first, rather than metformin, but metformin has other benefits and so could be co-prescribed from the start in this situation. The sulphonylurea is titrated upwards according to fasting blood glucose levels if available, or HbA1c. Such patients may need insulin adding early on, and their condition should be monitored closely.

Patients starting oral hypoglycaemic therapy in the UK are eligible for free prescriptions.

Second line

If the HbA1c is still not on target after 2–3 months, offer a second agent (see Table 7.1). Pioglitazone should be avoided in those with, or at risk of, heart failure, and in those at higher risk of bladder cancer. There is a tendency to avoid using it with older patients for these reasons. The short-acting sulphonylurea gliclazide can be given at a dose of 40–320 mg per day (if the slow release version is used, 30–120 mg). Doses above 160 mg should be given as two divided doses. If the patient is unwell, or actually losing weight, then insulin should be started without delay. This may also be appropriate if the HbA1c is still very high (e.g. over 75 mmol/mol).

Pioglitazone

Pioglitazone is very effective at reducing blood glucose, particularly in insulin-resistant patients, although it takes weeks or months to achieve its full effect. For this reason, a person whose Hba1c is responding but not at target after three months may simply need longer at the same dose rather than escalation of therapy. Pioglitazone has been found *not* to cause the increased risk of myocardial infarction that was a problem with rosiglitazone. However, there are numerous problems associated with the drug, which clinicians and patients should be aware of.

It can cause fluid retention and, therefore, can precipitate heart failure in susceptible individuals. This effect is greater when the drug is used with insulin. It should be avoided in people with significant liver disease, and has been associated with an increased risk of distal fractures in women. In 2011, it was found based on observational studies to be associated with a slightly increased risk of bladder cancer.

Although the risk of fluid retention is greater when insulin is co-prescribed, there is a place for pioglitazone in insulin-resistant patients taking high doses of insulin, provided the risks are justified and the patient is monitored closely for fluid retention.

Despite all of these problems, there is still a place for pioglitazone, and some patients may avoid starting insulin by using this drug. Such patients may accept some of the risks.

Careful patient selection is important. The drug is used less often now in older patients, as most of these problems become commoner with rising age. In younger patients at low risk of heart failure and of bladder cancer and no history of liver disease, it may be a useful way of reducing Hba1c. It should only be continued in patients who respond to it, and the benefits and risks should be discussed with the patient and reviewed periodically.

Third line

'Triple therapy' using metformin, a sulphonylurea, and either pioglitazone or a gliptin, is possible, but many patients using this combination are candidates for insulin, and this should always be considered before starting a third oral drug. Patients starting insulin can continue their oral medication, but an intensive insulin

---

Box 7.1 **Metformin**

Metformin is now the only available biguanide. Earlier drugs in this group included phenformin, which was withdrawn in the 1970s as it caused lactic acidosis. The biguanides are related to galegine, which was originally derived from the French lilac. This plant had been used for centuries to treat the symptoms of diabetes. Metformin is less lipophilic and safer than phenformin, rarely causing lactic acidosis, but is contraindicated in renal failure (see Chapter 13) for this reason. Metformin has a number of beneficial actions in diabetes. It reduces hepatic gluconeogenesis, increases insulin sensitivity and reduces carbohydrate absorption from the gastrointestinal tract. It also improves circulating free fatty acids and very low density lipoprotein (VLDL) levels. The UKPDS study suggested that metformin improves cardiovascular risk independently of its effect on blood glucose levels. Very occasionally, metformin causes reduction in vitamin B12 absorption, and serum B12 levels should be checked in patients taking metformin who develop peripheral neuropathy.

Box 7.2 **Advice on Gradual Introduction of Metformin to Avoid Side Effects**

Initiating metformin therapy (ADA/EASD advice):

1 Begin with low-dose metformin (500 mg) taken once or twice per day with meals (breakfast and/or dinner).
2 After 5–7 days, if gastrointestinal side-effects have not occurred, advance dose to 850 or 1000 mg before breakfast and dinner.
3 If GI side effects appear as doses advance, can decrease to previous lower dose and try to advance the dose at a later time.
4 The maximum effective dose is usually 850 mg twice per day, with modestly greater effectiveness with doses up to 3 g per day. GI side effects may limit the dose that can be used.
5 Based on cost considerations, generic metformin is the first choice of therapy. A longer-acting formulation is available and can be given once per day.

Table 7.1 Major classes of hypo-glycaemic agents and their current role in therapy.

Drug class and mode of action	Examples	Advantages	Disadvantages	Place in management
Biguanides: Reduces hepatic gluconeogenesis Increases insulin sensitivity Reduces carbohydrate absorption from the GI tract	Metformin is the only example in use	Weight neutral No risk of hypoglycaemia Possible cardiovascular benefits beyond hypoglycaemic effects Inexpensive	Gastrointestinal side-effects limit its usefulness	First line in the majority of patients, particularly those with insulin resistance
Sulphonylureas: Increase endogenous insulin production	Gliclazide Glimepiride Glibenclamide	Generally well tolerated Inexpensive Effective at reducing HbA1c and blood glucose in symptomatic patients	Risk of hypoglycaemia Weight gain	Usually second line in patients uncontrolled on metformin alone, but can be used alone in those unable to tolerate metformin or patients who are insulin-deficient
Glitazones: Increase tissue sensitivity to insulin	Pioglitazone is now the only example in use	Usually well tolerated May be used in combination with other oral therapies and with insulin	Take up to 12 weeks for maximum effect Risk of distal fractures in women May cause fluid retention and so precipitate heart failure in susceptible individuals Small degree of weight gain Small increased risk of bladder cancer, but benefits may outweigh risk in selected individuals	Usually second line in patients wishing to avoid the more significant weight gain with sulphonylureas, or third line in those still inadequately controlled on two agents (but insulin should be considered in such cases)
Incretin mimetics: Increase the release of endogenous insulin following carbohydrate ingestion Reduce release of pancreatic glucagon Delay gastric emptying Reduce calorie intake through central appetite suppression	Exenatide Liraglutide Lixisenatide	Actually reduce weight Can be used with either metformin, a sulphonylurea, or both	Injectable Relatively expensive Use with sulphonylurea substantially increases risk of hypoglycaemia Nausea and vomiting is common	Could be used as second line in a patient wishing to avoid weight gain, but can also be added in to a combination of metformin and sulphonylurea
DPP-4 Inhibitors: Delay the clearance of natural incretins	Sitagliptin Vildagliptin Linagliptin Saxagliptin	Weight neutral Sitagliptin can be used as triple therapy with metformin and a sulphonylurea	Relatively expensive	Can be added in second or third line
Meglitinides: Stimulate the release of pre-formed endogenous insulin	Repaglinide Nateglinide	Specifically aimed at post-prandial hyperglycaemia Rapid action	Multiple doses required before each meal Some risk of hypo	Repaglinide may be used as monotherapy Nateglinide only licensed for use with metformin
Alpha-glucosidase inhibitors: Delay the digestion and absorption of ingested carbohydrate	Acarbose	Reduces post-prandial hyperglycaemia Weight neutral	Poorly tolerated due to gastrointestinal side-effects including flatulence	Can be used alone or in combination with metformin and/or sulphonylurea
SGLT-2 inhibitors	Dapagliflozin Canagliflozin Empagliflozin	Do not in itself increase risk of hypoglycaemia (but could precipitate hypo if added to other therapies that do)	May increase risk of genital and urinary tract infection	Can be used as monotherapy if metformin not tolerated, or added to other therapies, including insulin if needed
Insulin therapy: Direct effect on tissues (particularly muscle and liver) to increase uptake of glucose from plasma	See Chapter 8	Effective at reducing HbA1c	Weight gain and need for high doses in insulin-resistant patients Require regular injection or a pump Risk of hypoglycaemia	Usually commenced when two oral agents have failed to achieve target, but should be considered wherever there are features of insulin deficiency, if control is very poor, or during intercurrent illness, to maintain control

therapy regimen may be simpler if the sulphonylurea is withdrawn, as the insulin is providing a similar effect exogenously. Most type 2 patients should continue taking metformin unless they fail to tolerate it or develop renal impairment. The patient who is actually *gaining* weight needs more dietary advice. Insulin and sulphonylureas tend to promote weight gain, and the injectable GLP-1 analogues may be useful in this situation. They stimulate glucose-mediated insulin secretion and so do not, on their own, cause hypoglycaemia. However, the risk of sulphonylurea-induced hypoglycaemia is substantially increased by concomitant GLP-1 (or gliptin) therapy. See Chapter 20 for more on its mode of action. Lixisenatide is licensed for use with basal insulin.

Other drug therapies

Other treatment options include the meglitinides (repaglinide or nateglinide), which are taken before a meal to promote insulin secretion and reduce post-prandial hyperglycaemia. Repaglinide is not recommended for use in patients over 75 years old. The alpha-glucosidase inhibitor *acarbose* acts by delaying carbohydrate absorption, and can be taken with other agents, but it is not well tolerated due to its gastrointestinal effects. Sodium Glucose Linked Transporter-2 (SGLT-2) inhibitors block the reabsorption of glucose in the kidney, lowering the blood glucose. By causing glycosuria they raise the risk of urinary tract infections, but may be useful in selected patients.

Cost-effectiveness and other considerations

Treatment choices may be guided by other issues, including cost and patient choice. All type 2 patients who can tolerate it should be offered metformin, which is inexpensive and very widely prescribed. Insulin therapy is generally the most effective option in terms of HbA1c reduction, but sulphonylureas are cheaper. For those taking a sulphonylurea who drive a car, self-monitoring at times relevant to driving is advised (Figure 7.2), and this adds to the cost. Pioglitazone is now also inexpensive but, unlike the latter, will not cause hypoglycaemia. This is also an advantage of GLP-1 analogues and the gliptins, unless they are co-prescribed with a sulphonylurea. Any patient taking a sulphonylurea may be at risk of hypo when a further drug is added, even if the new drug is not directly responsible. Table 7.1 describes some of the advantages and disadvantages of the individual agents.

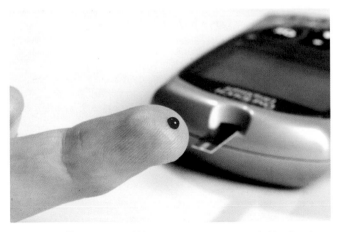

Figure 7.2 Self-monitoring of blood glucose is recommended in all patients taking insulin and may be justified in others on an individual basis.

Starting insulin in general practice

Insulin can be started in most type 2 patients in general practice. As described in Chapter 9, the usual preferred regimen is a twice daily dose of premixed insulin such as Novomix 30, given before breakfast and before the evening meal. It is usual to start at 6–8 u twice a day with home blood glucose monitoring. The monitoring technique should be taught prior to commencing (and not at the same time as) the insulin. The insulin can then be prescribed, and a new appointment arranged to demonstrate the injection technique. In addition to the insulin device, needles (usually 5 or 6 mm long), and a sharps disposal bin should be issued as repeat prescriptions. Needle-clipping devices are also prescribable and reduce the volume of sharps requiring disposal. Patients need to be clear about disposal arrangements for their sharps bins when full.

The insulin dose can be titrated upwards according to blood glucose levels, usually in increments of 2–4 units, as described in Chapter 9. An alternative is to start with a long-acting analogue such as glargine or detemir at eight units in the evening, titrating upwards according to fasting glucose levels. Conversion to a more flexible regimen can be achieved later on, either through the addition of short- or rapid-acting insulins with meals to create a basal-bolus regimen, or by changing over to a pre-mixed insulin twice or three times a day. By this time, the patient will have become accustomed to injections, and any initial needle phobia will have hopefully been overcome. The initial management of a once-daily long-acting analogue can usually be managed by general practice teams. Diabetes Specialist Nurses linked to the local hospital diabetes centre are very useful as a source of advice, guidance and patient education, particularly when insulin regimens become more complicated.

Unlike type 1 diabetes, type 2 is a progressive condition, in which insulin requirements are likely to increase over time. This should be borne in mind when selecting appropriate intervals to review adequacy of control.

Hypoglycaemia

As discussed in Chapter 10, hypoglycaemia may be seriously detrimental to quality of life and employment prospects. Type 2 patients starting insulin for the first time may or may not have experienced hypoglycaemia before (usually because of sulphonylureas). The risk of this happening is substantially greater with insulin and, in some cases, this may influence the decision to start insulin over other options, as discussed above. Patients should be counselled over the risk of hypo and given not only practical advice about how to correct it, but also a supply of glucagel and glucagon to be used if needed. Risk of hypoglycaemia is the main reason why those taking insulin (unless such treatment is only temporary – i.e. less than three months) are legally obliged to inform the Driver and Vehicle Licensing Agency (DVLA). Advice to inform the DVLA should be recorded in the notes. DVLA regulations are revised from time to time, and the latest guidance should be consulted.

Difficulties in achieving targets

Despite concerns about over-treatment, the reality is that too few patients manage to achieve their target HbA1c. In the UKPDS study, it was difficult to achieve and maintain control of glycaemia

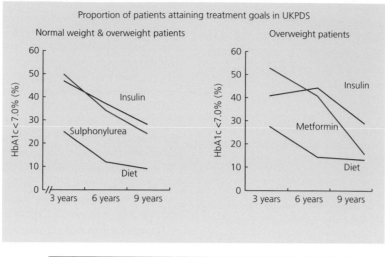

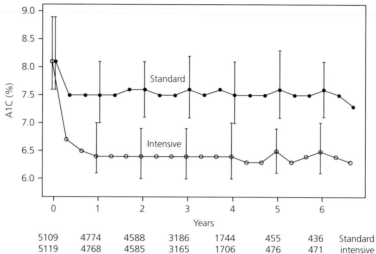

Figure 7.3 Proportion of patients attaining treatment goals in UKPDS. Source: Turner et al. (1999). Reproduced with permission of JAMA.

despite close supervision of trial participants (Figure 7.3a). However, in the later ACCORD study, partly through the advent of new drug options developed since UKPDS, tight control was maintained in the intensive treatment arm (Figure 7.3b). In real-world practice, this is difficult to achieve.

Further reading and references

Bailey CJ, Day C (2008). Glycaemic memory. *British Journal of Diabetes and Vascular Disease* **8**, 242–247.

Gaede P, Lund-Andersen H, Parving HH, Pedersen O (2008). Effect of a multifactorial intervention on mortality in type 2 diabetes. *New England Journal of Medicine* **358**, 580–591.

Gerstein HC, Miller ME, Byington RP et al.; Action to Control Cardiovascular Risk in Diabetes Study Group (2008). Effects of Intensive Glucose Lowering in Type 2 Diabetes. *New England Journal of Medicine* **358**, 2545–2559.

National Institute for Health and Clinical Governance (2009). *Type 2 diabetes – newer agents: short guideline.* Clinical Guideline No. 87, May 2009.

Nissen SE, Wolski K (2007). Effect of rosiglitazone on the risk of myocardial infarction and death from cardiovascular causes. *New England Journal of Medicine* **356**, 2457.

Turner RC, Cull CA, Frighi V, Holman RR (1999). Glycemic control with diet, sulfonylurea, metformin, or insulin in patients with type 2 diabetes mellitus: progressive requirement for multiple therapies. United Kingdom Prospective Diabetes (UKPDS) Group (49). *JAMA* **281**, 2005–2012.

Witters LA (2001). The blooming of the French lilac. *Journal of Clinical Investigation* **108**, 1105–1107.

CHAPTER 8

Hyperglycaemic Emergencies and Management of Diabetes in Hospital

Sailesh Sankar[1], Sudhesh Kumar[2] and Tim Holt[3]

[1]WISDEM, University Hospital Coventry and Warwickshire, Coventry, UK
[2]Warwick Medical School, University of Warwick; and WISDEM, University Hospital, Coventry, UK
[3]Nuffield Department of Primary Care Health Sciences, Oxford University, UK

OVERVIEW

- Hyperglycaemic emergencies include diabetic ketoacidosis (DKA) and hyperosmolar hyperglycaemic syndrome (HHS).

- Both require immediate treatment in hospital with insulin and fluid replacement.

- In DKA, the associated acidosis leads to loss of total body potassium, requiring close monitoring and intravenous potassium replacement during rehydration.

- Hyperviscosity may lead to thrombosis, particularly in older patients with HHS.

- Following recovery, patients require review of the treatment regimen and close follow-up to prevent recurrence.

- Patients admitted to hospital for elective procedures should be managed according to readily available protocols in order to optimise outcomes.

- Involvement of the diabetes specialist team is important when problems arise in hospitalised patients.

Introduction

A patient with severe hyperglycaemia can appear to be relatively well, so that potentially life-threatening diabetic ketoacidosis (DKA) or hyperosmolar hyperglycaemic syndrome (HHS) may go unrecognised. Thus, although a patient with significant hyperglycaemia can often be managed quite successfully out of hospital by experienced clinicians, if in doubt it is best to err on the safe side and send the patient to hospital.

Preventing diabetic ketoacidosis (DKA)

When a patient with diabetes presents with an acute illness, one should always assess the glycaemic control. During intercurrent infection, it is necessary for the patient to take larger doses of insulin than usual. Patients are usually taught this, but they often require support, especially if they have not dealt with a similar situation before. Often, while taking antibiotics, patients may have lost appetite and may feel that, as they are eating less, they should take less insulin. Unfortunately, some patients even stop insulin altogether during illness, and this is very likely to lead to diabetic ketoacidosis. If the patient is unable to eat or drink then, clearly, intravenous fluids and insulin will be required and the patient needs to go to hospital. However, for those patients who are managing an illness at home, regular frequent blood glucose monitoring and additional insulin should be taken, as informed by the blood glucose monitoring results. For those taking twice daily pre-mixed insulin, short-acting insulin is valuable if taken additionally.

Patients who have had diabetic ketoacidosis may also have been given blood or urine ketone meters or ketosticks. These are useful for indicating the onset of ketoacidosis. Sometimes ketoacidosis may be a presenting feature of type 1 diabetes or, rarely, late in type 2 diabetes.

Clinical features of ketoacidosis

Dehydration and tachypnoea are frequently seen early in DKA. Some clinicians may be able to smell ketone odour on the patient's breath. In more severe DKA, vomiting and drowsiness also develop.

Diagnosis

Blood glucose is typically very high but is sometimes only modestly raised, especially when the patient has not been eating regularly. In these cases, it is important to recognise that the degree of hyperglycaemia is not an index for the severity of the condition. Urine tests for ketones will be positive and plasma ketones will be elevated. Blood gases will show acidosis and reduced bicarbonate; blood ketones will reveal ketosis. Diabetic ketoacidosis is associated with severe electrolyte abnormalities, particularly of serum potassium. Electrolytes will need to be monitored frequently during the

ABC of Diabetes, Seventh Edition. Tim Holt and Sudhesh Kumar.
© 2015 John Wiley & Sons, Ltd. Published 2015 by John Wiley & Sons, Ltd.

treatment of DKA, as there is a net whole-body deficit of potassium. Potassium replacement is essential and guided by frequent electrolyte measurements.

Full blood counts will usually reveal leukocytosis which, however, does not necessarily imply infection. Similarly, serum amylase is often elevated but does not necessarily indicate pancreatitis. Further investigations are guided by additional clinical features of the particular patient. A chest x-ray is often carried out to exclude a chest infection. Urine analysis and urine culture may be required to exclude urinary tract infection. Blood culture may also be indicated if septicaemia is suspected. The need for further imaging is determined by the clinical presentation. In women of childbearing age, a pregnancy test should be carried out.

Treatment

Patients with diabetic ketoacidosis require high-intensity nursing on a one-to-one basis, and this is usually achieved in a High Dependency Unit or, if extremely ill and requiring ventilation, in an ITU setting. Factors suggesting the need for HDU care are given in Table 8.1.

Fluid and electrolyte management is key to successful treatment of DKA. This is achieved using intravenous saline; see Figure 8.1 for a suitable regimen. Care should be taken in patients with cardiac disease and post-myocardial infarction. In such patients, a central venous line and monitoring of central venous pressure (CVP) will be required. Once blood glucose drops below 14 mmol/l, 10% dextrose should be commenced alongside 0.9% saline, to enable more insulin to be administered intravenously to resolve the ketosis. Insulin is administered intravenously through a syringe driver in a fixed dose of 0.1 units per kilogram body weight. If the patient is on a basal insulin analogue, such as glargine or insulin detemir, this may be continued alongside the insulin infusion, enabling smoother transition to subcutaneous insulin regime during recovery. It is important that nursing staff check the equipment regularly, as kinks in the line for the fluids or insulin can complicate therapy.

Potassium replacement is nearly always required in patients with DKA, with the possible exception of patients who have advanced renal disease. Regular urea and electrolyte measurements should be requested, and potassium should be maintained between

Table 8.1 Factors suggesting the need for High Dependency Unit care.

The presence of one or more of these may require High Dependency Unit (HDU) care and immediate senior review

Blood ketones	>6 mmol/l
Venous bicarbonate	<5 mmol/l
Venous pH	<7.1
Hypokalaemia	<3.5 mmol/l on admission
GCS	<12
Oxygen saturation	<92% on air
Systolic blood pressure	<90 mm Hg
Pulse	>100 or < 60 beats per minute
Anion gap	>16
Pregnancy	
Heart failure	
Renal failure	
Other serious co-morbidities	

4–5 mmol/l as shown in the attached protocol. Tools are available for guiding management of fluid and potassium replacement (see Figure 8.2).

The acidosis usually corrects itself with fluid replacement and insulin. It is rarely necessary to give bicarbonate, except to buy time when the patient has life-threatening acidosis (pH < 6.9). When used, 1.26% bicarbonate should be given in 500 ml, and specialist supervision is recommended.

Insulin infusion should be continued until the patient is ready to eat and, ideally, ketosis is resolved. At this point, the patient should be given subcutaneous insulin and, after the meal, IV insulin is discontinued. One should aim to ensure that ketosis has resolved (ketones < 0.6 mmol/l, venous pH > 7.3), and that bicarbonate is > 18 mmol/l before discharge.

The underlying condition needs to be sought and treated, and sick day rules (see Chapter 11, Box 11.5) should be reinforced to the patient to avoid the same occurring again.

'Brittle diabetes'

A small number of patients have very unstable diabetes that completely disrupts their lives, with repeated admissions to hospital due to either DKA or hypoglycaemia. It is more common in young girls. Often, there are underlying psychological issues that can be quite challenging to manage.

Mismatch of the dose of insulin, relative to the patient's diet or exercise, should be dealt with. Patients may benefit from learning the technique of carbohydrate counting. Further education through the DAFNE (Dose Adjustment For Normal Eating) programme is also helpful in some cases (see Chapters 3 and 11). If this does not resolve the problem, some of these patients will benefit from continuous subcutaneous insulin infusion through an insulin pump. This requires specialist assessment and management and such patients should be referred to hospital.

Hyperosmolar hyperglycaemic syndrome

These patients often have an extremely high degree of hyperglycaemia without significant acidosis or ketosis. The term 'hyperosmolar hyperglycaemic syndrome' (HHS) is now used in preference to 'hyperosmolar non-ketotic' (HONK), to recognise that a mild degree of ketosis may be present. Significant ketonaemia (>3 mmol/l and acidosis (pH < 7.3) are features of DKA rather than HHS. The management is similar to that of DKA, with intravenous fluid and insulin replacement, but such patients often require prophylactic subcutaneous heparin to prevent thrombotic complications.

The patient should be rehydrated by at least 2–3 litres by six hours, and hyperglycaemia should be corrected by insulin infusion in addition to fluids. They are less likely to require potassium replacement during rehydration. If hyperosmolarity is so severe that serum sodium is greater than 150, half normal saline is used until serum sodium is below 150 mmol/l. Although the biochemical abnormalities in HHS are less complex than in DKA, the condition carries a higher mortality (≈15% compared to < 5%). As in DKA, the precipitating cause should be identified and treated.

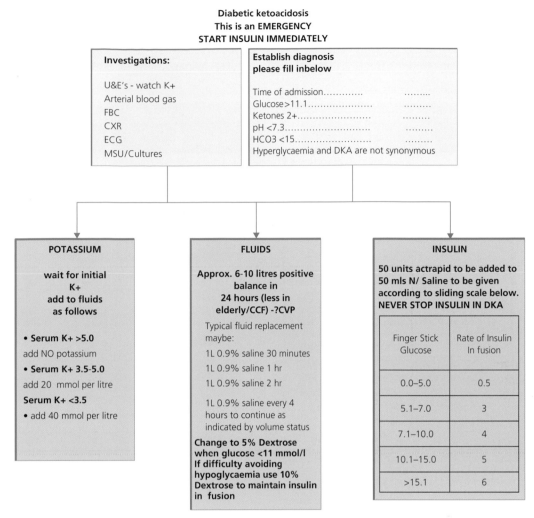

Figure 8.1 Protocol for the hospital management of diabetic ketoacidosis used at the University Hospital, Coventry.

Management of hospitalised type 2 diabetic patients

The management of a type 2 diabetic patient admitted for elective surgery is usually quite straightforward, so long as the patient is well controlled. All that is needed is to omit the oral hypoglycaemic agent on the day of surgery, and to monitor plasma glucose. If plasma glucose is greater than 11 mmol/l in the morning, IV soluble insulin via an insulin pump will be required.

For patients undergoing relatively minor surgery, so long as the operation is done first thing in the morning and the patient is able to eat and drink within a hour of the procedure, this can be accomplished without the need for hospital admission. In this case, it is important that the patient is able to self-manage their diabetes soon after the procedure. Protocols used at the University Hospital, Coventry are shown in Figure 8.1.

Management of diabetes for major elective surgery and type 1 diabetic patients

Management of patient with diabetes for elective surgery should be planned and control should be optimised before the surgery. It is recommended that the patient be referred to the diabetes specialist team for advice if HbA1c is greater than 69 mmol/mol (8.5%).

Such operations are usually managed by intravenous insulin, administered using an infusion pump. Use 0.45% sodium chloride and 5% glucose, with either 0.15% or 0.3% potassium chloride (as appropriate) as the substrate fluid of choice if a VRIII is required. Consider continuation of long-acting analogues (Glargine/Lantus®, Detemir/Levemir®) alongside the VRIII during the peri-operative period. Maintain blood glucose level between 6–10 mmol/l where possible.

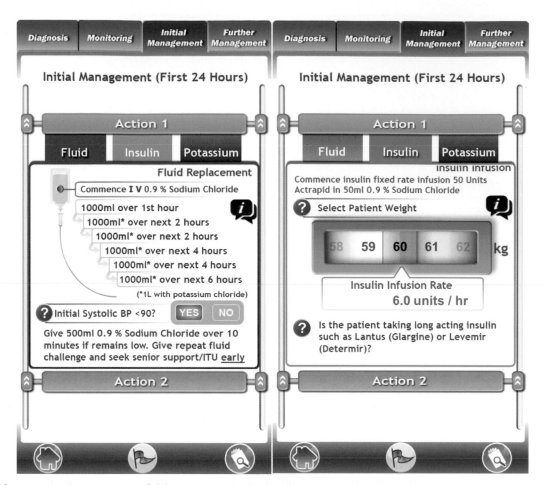

Figure 8.2 Tool for supporting the management of diabetic emergencies developed by Domz Creations (http://domzcreations.com/). Source: Domz Creations.

Regular monitoring of plasma glucose is required, and electrolytes should also be measured at least once a day. If blood glucose levels are consistently above 12 mmol/l for three consecutive times, the rate of insulin infusion will have to be reviewed.

In patients with type 1 diabetes, it is important to remember that intravenous insulin should not be stopped, as such patients can deteriorate very rapidly. Circulating plasma insulin levels decay rapidly if there is no subcutaneous reserve. Conversion to the usual insulin regime should be made only when the patient is able to eat and drink normally. Once the subcutaneous insulin injection has been given and the patient has had a meal, the IV insulin can be discontinued. If the patient is hyperglycaemic after conversion to subcutaneous insulin, additional soluble insulin can be given, but care should be taken to avoid hypoglycaemia at the same time.

The role of technology in improving inpatient diabetes care

Inpatient diabetes care is now a new focus on quality indicators. Care of patients with diabetes during their inpatient stay is complex, and compounded by the fact that the majority of them are not necessarily under a specialist diabetes team. Often, the primary reason for their admission is unrelated to their diabetes, but various interventions and physiological and pathological stress have an impact on their diabetes.

Use of technology can further enhance improving care. Systems and software exist to enable blood glucose monitoring data to be wirelessly transferred to a diabetes data management system and, hence, enable health professionals to proactively institute changes. Electronic prescribing can further enhance patient safety and reduce insulin errors. Mobile apps and devices can also aid in improving patient safety during their inpatient stay. An example of such an app is iDKA (free download from iTunes) to aid health professional manage patients with diabetic ketoacidosis. The future of inpatient diabetes care can be improved by embracing newer technologies and incorporating them with improved training and education of staffs and patients.

Further reading

American Diabetes Association (2004). Hyperglycemic crises in diabetes. *Diabetes Care* **27**, S94–S102.

Cook CB, Zimmerman RS, Gauthier SM (2008). Understanding and Improving Management of Inpatient Diabetes Mellitus: The Mayo Clinic Arizona Experience. *Journal of Diabetes Science and Technology* **2**(6), 925–931.

JBDS 02. *The Hospital Management of DKA in Adults*. Revised September 2013.

JBDS 03. *The management of adults with diabetes undergoing surgery and elective procedures: improving standards*. April 2011.

JBDS 06. *The management of the hyperosmolar hyperglycaemic state (HHS) in adults with diabetes*. August 2012.

Scott A (2006). Hyperosmolar hyperglycaemic syndrome. *Diabetic Medicine* **23**(Suppl. 3), 22–24.

Singh RK, Perros P, Frier BM (2004). Hospital management of diabetic ketoacidosis: are clinical guidelines implemented effectively? *Diabetic Medicine* **14**, 482–486.

CHAPTER 9

Insulin Therapy

Tim Holt[1] and Sudhesh Kumar[2]

[1]Nuffield Department of Primary Care Health Sciences, Oxford University, UK
[2]Warwick Medical School, University of Warwick; and WISDEM, University Hospital, Coventry, UK

OVERVIEW

- Patients presenting with type 1 diabetes require insulin without delay to avoid ketoacidosis.

- An increasing proportion of type 2 patients will require insulin to achieve modern glycaemic control targets.

- The majority of type 2 patients requiring insulin can have this treatment initiated in primary care.

- A wide range of insulin types is available, but most patients can be managed using a limited selection of regimens and devices.

- Familiarity with these devices and regimens overcomes the inertia that may delay the initiation of insulin in type 2 diabetes.

- Insulin pumps are becoming an increasingly available means of optimizing glycaemic control.

Introduction

Insulin replacement therapy is essential for a patient with type 1 diabetes, and is needed to achieve good glycaemic control in many patients with type 2 diabetes once other agents are no longer able to achieve this effectively. For patients with previously poor glycaemic control, insulin has dramatic effects, and it can enhance wellbeing in a way that other therapies cannot match. Despite these obvious benefits, many patients who have previously taken tablets resist going onto insulin therapy, principally because it is an injectable preparation. Insulin therapy also requires much more active involvement by the patient to adjust the doses.

Insulin is unusual as a drug in that the dose different patients take may range very widely, from a few units to several hundred units. This often makes healthcare professionals with limited experience wary of managing patients on insulin. The optimal dose is tailored for every given patient, and is one that achieves the best possible control, avoiding hypoglycaemia as much as possible. In older, frailer patients, it might be inappropriate to provide intensive insulin therapy, and here a once-daily insulin injection that alleviates the symptoms may be all that is required.

Types of insulin

1 *Animal insulins*. Until the 1980s, insulin was manufactured from purified extracts from the pancreas of cows and pigs. Today, it is manufactured by recombinant DNA technology that involves the insertion of the synthesised genes for insulin into *Escherichia coli* bacteria, or yeast cells. The resulting protein is yielded in large quantities, then purified. Some patients still use animal insulin – often those individuals who experienced hypoglycaemia after commencing human insulin. Today, the vast majority of people with diabetes in the UK use human insulin.

2 *Short-acting insulins*. Short-acting insulin is also known as soluble insulin. It has a duration of action of about 6-8 hours and needs to be injected about 30 minutes before meals. Examples are listed in Table 9.1.

3 *Very rapid-acting insulin analogues*. These are newer human insulin analogues that can be taken with, or just after, a meal, because they are absorbed more or less immediately. They are used to cover mealtime carbohydrate intake in a basal-bolus insulin regime, which is discussed later.

4 *Intermediate-acting insulins*. These insulins usually have a basic protein such as protoamine, or zinc, added to them to delay their action. They generally tend to have a duration of action of about 8-10 hours after subcutaneous injection. Variants are also available, where a duration of action that is considerably longer can be obtained.

5 *Long-acting insulin zinc suspensions*. These are prepared by adding excess zinc ions to insulin; examples include ultratard and humulin zinc. These are usually administered at bedtime.

6 *Long-acting insulin analogues*. These insulin analogues provide up to 24-hour basal insulin when injected subcutaneously. Such preparations may be suitable for once-daily administration, and they carry a low-risk of hypoglycaemia because their action profile does not have a prominent 'peak', unlike short-acting or intermediate-acting insulins.

7 *Pre-mixed insulin mixtures*. Several preparations of insulin are available as pre-prepared mixtures in vials, or as pre-mixed pens, eliminating the need for patients to mix insulin in a syringe. This

ABC of Diabetes, Seventh Edition. Tim Holt and Sudhesh Kumar.
© 2015 John Wiley & Sons, Ltd. Published 2015 by John Wiley & Sons, Ltd.

Table 9.1 Commonly used types of insulin, with examples.

Type of insulin	Examples	Comments
Soluble insulin	Human Actrapid, Pork Actrapid, Humulin S	Actrapid now only available in vials
Rapid-acting insulin analogues	Aspart (Novorapid), Lispro (Humalog), Glulisine (Apidra)	Onset only takes 15 minutes so can be given immediately after, rather than before, a meal, when the exact carbohydrate intake is known, if this suits the patient. Short duration of action reduces risk of nocturnal hypoglycaemia and provides flexibility for dose adjustment. Risk of overlap with subsequent injection later in the day is reduced.
Long-acting insulin analogues	Glargine (Lantus), Detemir (Levemir), Degludec (Tresiba).	Have little or no 'peak' of action and are, therefore, useful as the basal component of the basal-bolus regimen. Degludec is a new, ultra-long acting formulation that has been shown to provide similar control of Hba1c, with reduction in risk of hypoglycaemia in type 1 diabetes.
Isophane (NPH)	Insulatard, Humulin I, Insuman Basal, Hypurin Porcine Isophane, Hypurin Bovine Isophane	Still used as the basal component, but does 'peak' in its action. This effect may be useful, but may contribute to the risk of nocturnal hypoglycaemia. Significantly less expensive than long-acting analogues
Biphasic 'pre-mixed' insulins or insulin analogues	Biphasic insulin aspart (Novomix 30), Biphasic insulin Lispro (Humalog Mix25 and Mix50), Mixtard (10, 20, 30, 40, 50), Humulin M3, Insuman Comb (15, 25, 50)	Useful for patients requiring some flexibility but wishing to avoid the more intensive basal-bolus regimen (which requires at least four injections a day). Can be given twice or three times a day before meals. The proportion of overall insulin in the soluble form is indicated by the number. A commonly used option is the '30' strength

reduces the risk of mistakes made while mixing insulin, and is also more convenient. Examples of popular insulin mixtures are shown in Table 9.1. The choice of a mixture is dependent on the patient's lifestyle and meal patterns. Similarly, the selection of particular insulins for a patient is also made bearing in mind the patient's particular circumstances, and also their preferences in terms of choice of device and frequency of injection.

Insulin regimens

Starting insulin in type 1 diabetes

Many type 1 patients can start treatment with a twice-daily biphasic regimen – usually about eight units twice a day – and then the dose is optimised. However, in younger patients in particular, a more flexible method is the basal-bolus regime, where a long-acting insulin is given at bedtime and meals are covered by soluble insulin or a very short-acting analogue. An increasing number of people in the UK now use insulin analogues, especially if they experience hypoglycaemia on conventional insulins.

Basal-bolus regime

Here, an intermediate- or long-acting acting insulin is used at bedtime, and meals are covered using a short-acting insulin or a rapid-acting insulin analogue. A long-acting insulin analogue, such as insulin glargine or insulin detemir, is often used in the UK now as the basal insulin. However, twice-daily NPH insulin (which is intermediate acting) provides an effective basal component, and was the basal insulin used in the DAFNE trial discussed in Chapters 3 and 12. The timing of the rapid-acting insulin can vary according to the timing of meals, which is convenient for those at work or at college. Rapid-acting insulin analogues have made this regimen more popular, because they avoid the overlap effects that may cause problems with frequently administered soluble insulin.

Twice or three times a day biphasic regimen

Some patients opt to have twice-daily biphasic mixtures, taken at breakfast and with an evening meal. This can be increased by adding in a lunchtime dose if using a biphasic with a rapid-acting component, but there may in some cases be a risk of overlap between the lunchtime and evening doses. Occasionally, such patients may require a short-acting or rapid-acting insulin with lunch, instead of the biphasic.

Starting insulin in type 2 diabetes

For some type 2 patients, it may be appropriate simply to provide a once-daily insulin injection with a long-acting insulin analogue. This approach was shown in the 4T study to be associated with fewer hypos and less weight gain than prandial insulin alone or a biphasic regimen, when added in to oral therapy with metformin and a sulphonylurea. For many patients, however, pre-mixed insulin or an insulin analogue may provide more effective control of post-prandial glycaemia, as it contains a short- or rapid-acting component. Some patients with type 2 diabetes also elect to go on a basal bolus regimen, which involves four or more injections a day, because of the flexibility it offers. For many patients, a twice or three times a day regimen of pre-mixed analogues is useful.

Maintaining glycaemic control in a patient with type 2 diabetes represents more of a challenge, as their needs will change along with disease progression. The doses are increased usually in increments of two or four units with each dose, until glucose control is satisfactory, taking care to avoid hypoglycaemia. It is important to explain this to the patient, and also to alter insulin doses and the regime as requirements increase. Patients should also be warned about weight gain, particularly in those with type 2 diabetes, and concomitant attention to control of obesity is valuable in mitigating this. There is more discussion on insulin management of type 2 patients in Chapter 7.

Administering insulin

In the past, most patients used a syringe to draw up and administer insulin. The following modes of administration are now available:
1 *Insulin administered with a syringe*. The patient uses a syringe to draw the appropriate dose from a vial. These plastic insulin syringes are often still preferred by patients who have been using

them for years, but are less likely to be chosen by patients who start insulin today.

2 *Insulin 'pens'.* These are quite sophisticated and reliable devices, which deliver metered doses of insulin, either from a cartridge or as a pre-loaded disposable pen that is discarded once the insulin has been fully dispensed. Mixtard 30 is available as a 'InnoLet' device, which may be convenient for patients with visual or manual dexterity problems.

3 *Insulin pumps.* There are now several types of insulin pumps available, and the size has reduced so that they are quite unobtrusive. These pumps deliver insulin subcutaneously over 24 hours, and there are facilities for prandial boosts of insulin. Corrective dose requirements, based on carbohydrate intake and the current blood glucose level (entered by the patient), can be calculated by the device and delivered. Insulin pump therapy should be managed by secondary care centres that provide readily accessible expertise to handle any problems. Pump failure may rapidly lead to insulin deficiency, with risk of ketosis, as the formulation used is rapid-acting and has a short plasma half-life. Their use is restricted on the NHS to those who cannot be managed otherwise on basal-bolus therapy.

4 *Inhaled insulin.* Inhaled insulin was recently launched, but was unsuccessful and has since been withdrawn from the market, as it did not prove to be as popular as anticipated. Nevertheless, newer varieties of inhaled insulins are due on the market. These are of value, perhaps, only for those patients with severe needle-phobia.

Insulin injection sites

Sites that can be used for insulin injection are shown in Figure 9.1. It is most commonly injected in the front of the thigh, or on the lower abdominal wall. Patients are advised to rotate sites, to reduce the risk of unsightly bruises or fat hypertrophy. Injection sites should be inspected in case lipohypertrophy develops, as this can cause instability in glycaemic control, due to variable rates of absorption of insulin.

Insulin injection technique

When the patient first starts insulin, he or she is shown how to inject it using the device that has been chosen. The correct dose of insulin is drawn up using the pen, and any air bubbles are expelled prior to injection. The length of the needle will also have been

chosen for the given patient, and the needle should be inserted briskly, at 90° to the skin, to its whole length. Pressing the plunger rapidly will deliver the dose, and the device is then removed.

Problems with insulin injections

Apart from injection site bruises, insulin injections rarely cause problems. Occasionally, insulin allergy may appear and, in these cases, switching the type of insulin may help. In some cases, investigation by skin testing and desensitisation may be needed. Lipohypertrophy at injection sites may occur, and it is important to avoid injecting into these areas, as absorption is unreliable. Patients who have commenced insulin therapy sometimes experience blurring of vision, due to changes in the amount of water in the lens. This usually corrects itself in a few weeks, and the patients should be advised not to change their spectacle prescription during this time or to purchase new glasses. Oedema of the feet is also a transient phenomenon, and some patients with mild neuropathy may experience a worsening of pain in the feet when starting insulin. This, again, will improve with time.

Insulin pump therapy

For patients with type 1 diabetes above the age of 12 years with sub-optimal glycaemic control and/or disabling frequent episodes of hypoglycaemia, it is worth considering an insulin pump (Figure 9.2). This is a device that delivers insulin continuously throughout the day; it attempts to mimic the physiological release of insulin, but it is delivered subcutaneously. The insulin pump delivers insulin in two ways: a *basal* rate which is a continuous, background of subcutaneous insulin that keeps blood glucose stable between meals and overnight; and a *bolus* rate, which is added with meals to provide additional insulin to cover meals.

Suitable patients need further assessment by a specialist to consider whether the patient is able to comply with the requirements for living with a pump, and to understand how to adjust doses according to blood glucose readings. Sometimes, patients with poor awareness of hypoglycaemia are also provided a device to enable continuous monitoring of glucose, and with a set level at which an alarm is provided to alert the patient when hypoglycaemia has set

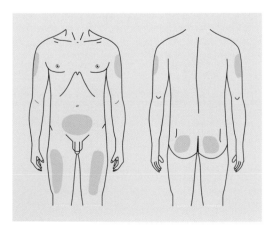

Figure 9.1 Injection sites.

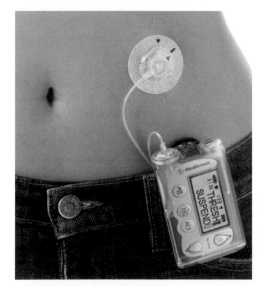

Figure 9.2 Insulin pump. Photograph: iStock. Source: eHealthyBlog.com

in. Main risks include injection site infections, and the rare occurrence of pump failure. The details of management of an insulin pump are out of the scope of this book, and referral to a specialist is advised for managing patients on insulin pumps

Summary

Insulin therapy should, where possible, be tailored to the needs and preferences of the individual, which differ widely across different patient groups. A need for flexibility is provided for by the rapid-acting insulin analogues that have proven extremely useful for intensive insulin management, where life-style patterns and schedules change from day to day. Long-acting insulin analogues have significantly improved the problem of nocturnal hypoglycaemia associated with 'peaking' of the older intermediate-acting insulins.

However, for many patients, the older insulins are very satisfactory, particularly where glycaemic control is not the main issue. For health services, there are cost implications with the newer formulations. Optimisation of glycaemic control should, however, be a health service priority, given the benefits both in terms of quality of life and avoidance of longer term complications.

Further reading

Bolli GB (2001). Physiological insulin replacement in type 1 diabetes mellitus. *Experimental and Clinical Endocrinology & Diabetes* **109**(Suppl. 2), S317–S332.

Gallichan M, O'Brien S, Dromgoole P, Nute B, Preston F, Tipson M (2004). *Starting insulin treatment in adults with type 2 diabetes*. Royal College of Nurses. http://www.rcn.org.uk/__data/assets/pdf_file/0009/78606/002254.pdf

Garber AJ, King AB, Del Prato S, Sreenan S, Balci MK, Muñoz-Torres M, Rosenstock J, Endahl LA, Francisco AM, Hollander P, NN1250-3582 (BEGIN BB T2D) Trial Investigators (2012). Insulin degludec, an ultra-longacting basal insulin, versus insulin glargine in basal-bolus treatment with mealtime insulin aspart in type 2 diabetes (BEGIN Basal-Bolus Type 2): a phase 3, randomised, open-label, treat-to-target non-inferiority trial. *Lancet* **379**(9825), 1498–1507.

Heller S, Buse J, Fisher M, Garg S, Marre M, Merker L, Renard E, Russell-Jones D, Philotheou A, Francisco AM, Pei H, Bode B, BEGIN Basal-Bolus Type 1 Trial Investigators (2012). Insulin degludec, an ultra-longacting basal insulin, versus insulin glargine in basal-bolus treatment with mealtime insulin aspart in type 1 diabetes (BEGIN Basal-Bolus Type 1): a phase 3, randomised, open-label, treat-to-target non-inferiority trial. *Lancet* **379**(9825), 1489–1497.

Holman RR, Farmer AJ, Davies MJ, Levy JC, Darbyshire JL, Keenan JF, Paul SK, for the 4-T Study Group (2009). Three-Year Efficacy of Complex Insulin Regimens in Type 2 Diabetes. *New England Journal of Medicine* **361**, 1736–1747.

Pickup J, Keen H (2001). Continuous subcutaneous insulin infusion in type 1 diabetes. *BMJ* **322**, 1262–1263.

Richter B, Neises G (2005). '*Human' insulin versus animal insulin in people with diabetes mellitus*. Cochrane Library. http://www.mrw.interscience.wiley.com/cochrane/clsysrev/articles/CD003816/frame.html.

CHAPTER 10

Hypoglycaemia

Tim Holt[1], Sudhesh Kumar[2] and Noreen Kumar[3]

[1]Nuffield Department of Primary Care Health Sciences, Oxford University, UK
[2]Warwick Medical School, University of Warwick; and WISDEM, University Hospital, Coventry, UK
[3]St James's Hospital, Leeds, UK

OVERVIEW

- Patients should aim to keep blood glucose levels above 3.9 mmol/l at all times.

- Tight glycaemic control increases the risk of hypoglycaemia.

- Common causes are too much insulin or sulphonylurea, missed meals or unexpected exercise.

- Symptoms may change over time and some may not perceive any symptoms.

- Steps should be taken to reduce risk of further episodes of hypoglycaemia by adjusting diet, activity or dose of insulin or sulphonylurea.

Introduction

Hypoglycaemic episodes are common and often go unrecognised, potentially leading to severe morbidity. This is most commonly seen in type 1 diabetes, but also occurs in type 2 patients, especially those taking sulphonylureas or insulin. Symptoms can occur at significantly higher blood glucose levels than the usual lower reference range limit of 3.5 mmol/l, particularly in those with long-standing poor glycaemic control. In some patients, the normal protective neurohormonal response to falling blood glucose levels is impaired, thus increasing the risk of hypoglycaemia.

Preventing the complications of diabetes is clearly important, and current treatment guidelines recommend near normoglycaemia for most patients. However, tight glycaemic control increases the risk of hypoglycaemia as much as threefold, and may be associated with altered cognitive function, seizures or coma. Thus, clinicians must balance the importance of tight control with the potential psychosocial effects that hypoglycaemia may have for the individual. Patients find hypoglycaemia distressing, and clinicians should temper their enthusiasm for achieving ideal HbA1c targets by recognising the difficulties that this may cause for some people. Treatment goals should be individually negotiated as part of the patient-centred approach.

Causes

Hypoglycaemia most commonly occurs as a result of inadvertent insulin or sulphonylurea overdose, or a change in dose. Other causes include a missed or inadequate meal, unexpected exercise, or an error in the timing of insulin. Due to the slow absorption and the mealtime peaks of insulin levels, the risk of hypoglycaemia is greatest:

- between meal times;
- in the middle of the night, when both soluble and intermediate-acting insulins may be having their peak effect. It may be helpful to reduce the pre-evening meal soluble insulin, and to move the evening intermediate-acting insulin to bedtime. It is essential that such patients have a bedtime snack. The use of rapid-acting insulin analogues rather than soluble insulin before meals make nocturnal hypoglycaemia less likely, particularly if teatime is several hours before sleep.

Recently diagnosed type 2 patients may experience episodes of hypoglycaemia several hours after meals. Symptoms in these patients are generally brief.

Some patients are concerned about possible increased hypoglycaemia with human insulin. This is often related to their experience following the switch in the early 1980s from using purified animal (mainly porcine) insulin to human insulin as the routine treatment of diabetes mellitus. Studies of human insulin have not shown any basis for concern that human insulin may cause harm in this way. However, high-quality research on patient-oriented outcomes such as quality of life is lacking.

Recognising the hypoglycaemic patient: the clinical picture

Typical symptoms experienced by adults occur as a result of the direct effects of glucose deprivation on the brain, causing neuroglycopenic symptoms such as confusion, drowsiness and difficulty concentrating. Autonomic symptoms result from simultaneous stimulation of the sympatho-adrenal system, leading to sweating, tremor and anxiety.

Table 10.1 Common symptoms of hypoglycaemia.

Common symptoms	
CNS	Headache, confusion, difficulty concentrating, personality changes
Cardiovascular	Palpitations
GI	Hunger, nausea, belching
Adrernergic	Sweating, anxiety

Table 10.2 Recognising those at risk of severe hypoglycaemia.

Risk factors for severe hypoglycaemia in diabetes mellitus
Type 1 diabetes with a history of recurrent severe hypoglycaemia
Young patients
Elderly patients on sulphonylureas
Alcohol
Strenuous exercise in past 24 hours
Critical illness such as sepsis, hepatic, renal or cardiac failure

At every visit, episodes attributed to hypoglycaemia should be discussed. Patients may also experience 'hypos' that go unrecognised. Symptoms are influenced by age. Behavioural changes, including lethargy, are common in children, while elderly patients are more likely to experience neurological effects such as visual disturbance, loss of balance and poor coordination. Table 10.1 lists some of the common symptoms.

Although these are the common presenting symptoms, each patient will learn to recognise their own hypoglycaemic episodes, as symptom profiles vary from patient to patient. Some may recognise that certain insulins result in greater hypoglycaemic effects. Table 10.2 highlights the patients at high risk of severe hypoglycaemia. Patients in these categories need greater vigilance, both in planning the antidiabetic regimen and the acute treatment of hypoglycaemia.

Hypoglycaemia unawareness

A very common problem, which rises in prevalence with increasing duration of diabetes, is the syndrome of 'impaired awareness of hypoglycaemia'. This is the lack of warning symptoms of prevailing hypoglycaemia, due to defective epinepherine release and reduced autonomic neural response normally accompanying hypoglycaemia. This condition occurs in about 25% of patients with long-standing disease, and is often the result of patients using intensified insulin therapy in order to achieve chronic normoglycaemia. Many of the classical symptoms are either reduced in intensity or lost altogether. This results in a diminished ability to recognise the onset of symptoms, leaving the patient with a significantly increased risk of severe neuroglycopenic hypoglycaemia. This manifests as sudden changes in personality, intellectual function or conscious level, without the patient's awareness.

Previous episodes of hypoglycaemia may predispose patients to further episodes. In some patients, it may be that their body no longer recognises low blood sugars as dangerous, and fails to mount a protective response until a more severe level of hypoglycaemia occurs. In these patients, a blood glucose level of less than 4.0 mmol/l should be meticulously avoided.

A clue to the patient with reduced hypoglycaemia awareness is a glycaemic profile that includes very low blood glucose measurements. If the patient frequently needs to check their level when it is less than 3.9 mmol/l, then it is likely that they have reduced awareness. Generally, if aware of the hypo the person should act immediately by taking rapidly absorbed glucose without delay. However, some may have been advised to take a measurement when hypoglycaemic to determine how low it has fallen. Clinicians have a duty to the rest of society, and hypoglycaemia unawareness is a serious development that needs to be 'risk managed' appropriately. If significant and likely to persist, it usually precludes safe driving, and the Driver and Vehicle Licensing Authority (DVLA) will need to be informed.

In some cases, changes to treatment with improved stability but higher average blood glucose levels may restore hypoglycaemia awareness, and the DVLA may then agree to resumption of driving. These decisions need to be openly discussed and well documented, in view of the legal implications.

Treatment of the acute episode in adults

Mild episodes can be self-treated by the patient, usually by taking a form of oral carbohydrate containing refined glucose. For example, mild episodes can be treated with glucose tablets or some other rapid-acting source of glucose.

All forms of refined sugar take approximately 10–15 minutes to relieve symptoms. This delay may result in persisting symptoms that commonly encourage over-treatment, resulting in subsequent hyperglycaemia and triggering a 'vicious cycle'. Symptomatic recovery of hypoglycaemia should be followed by ingestion of complex or unrefined carbohydrate, such as biscuits or breakfast cereal, in order to prevent recurrence of the hypoglycaemia. Vigorous exercise and driving should be avoided.

If hypoglycaemia occurs while the patient is driving, they should pull over and park the car at the earliest safe opportunity, switch the engine off, remove the keys from the ignition and move out of the driver seat. Driving should not resume until at least 45 minutes have elapsed *after the resumption of a recorded normal blood glucose level*, in view of the potential delay to the return of normal cognitive function.

Treatment of hypoglycaemia is related to duration and severity of the episode. Box 10.1 shows the emergency management of acute hypoglycaemia in adults (British National Formulary).

Glucagon can be used if the patient is at home or IV access cannot be rapidly obtained. In adults, 1 mg glucagon should be given by intramuscular or subcutaneous injection.

The cause of the hypoglycaemia should always be sought for every episode. The patient's current medication should be reviewed, and the appropriate adjustment of insulin dose or hypoglycaemic tablets should be made if necessary. The patient should be advised about common causes of hypoglycaemia, such as alcohol and exercise, and should also be educated about the importance of snacks between meals, as well as before and after exercise.

For type 1 patients, it may be easy to identify that a hypo has occurred as a result of a miscalculation in the amount of insulin required to balance carbohydrate intake and exercise. Changes in the regular doses may then be unnecessary, and the main lesson learned may concern the glycaemic effect of the particular carbohydrate

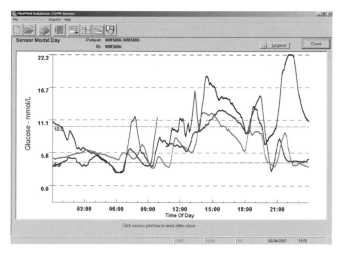

Figure 10.1 Three-day profile of glucose values sampled every five minutes from a patient using an insulin pump, with a different colour for each day, superimposed. This shows a risk of (or actual) hypoglycaemia early in the day, with generally higher values later. Source: Reproduced with permission of Medtronic.

source. In type 2 patients taking sulphonylureas, however, the occurrence of hypoglycaemia usually means that a reduction in dosage is appropriate.

Hypoglycaemia in children

Children may not have such dramatic symptoms when having a hypoglycaemic episode, but they may appear unduly lethargic.

Prompt treatment of hypoglycaemia is especially important in children to prevent any subsequent neurological damage. The parent should be advised that a hypoglycaemic episode that causes unconsciousness or fitting is a medical emergency. In the long term, parents, other carers and the child should be educated about how to recognise the onset of a hypoglycaemic episode. They should always have access to an immediate source of carbohydrate, and blood glucose monitoring equipment for immediate confirmation and management of the hypoglycaemia.

The child (depending on the age and ability) should be involved in the management of their condition, to ensure greater independence and confidence in the future. When children present with episodes of hypoglycaemia, it is particularly important to ensure that the child is taking the correct dose of insulin. If the child finds it hard to adhere to multiple daily injections, twice-daily injection regimens should be offered.

Long-term management of the patient

Greater emphasis on self-management may help patients control parameters that reduce the risk of hypoglycaemia. With the correct education and support, many patients can become expert at managing their disease, ensuring normoglycaemia and minimising the risk of hypoglycaemia. This may be achieved by:

- Basic education in the management of diabetes, with constant re-enforcement and support.
- A better understanding of concepts such as carbohydrate counting and self-adjustment of the dose of insulin may help

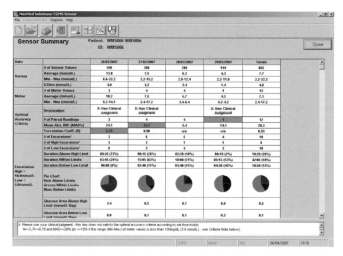

Figure 10.2 The same profile is automatically analysed to identify the proportion of values in range, or in the hypo- or hyperglycaemic ranges (pie chart), as well as mean values by day . Source: Reproduced with permission of Medtronic.

reduce risk of hypoglycaemia. The DAFNE programme is discussed in Chapters 3 and 11.

- Objective ways to monitor both the condition and the awareness of hypoglycaemia through blood glucose profiling. As well as traditional self-monitoring, this is now possible through continuous monitoring systems that sample glucose levels subcutaneously every few minutes (see Figures 10.1 and 10.2). However, these are usually only available through outpatient clinics on an occasional basis, and not for long-term use at the present time.
- Developing the skills to adjust the treatment regime when necessary. This may require protracted training with frequent review but, once achieved, it may be very empowering and of lasting benefit.

Further reading

British National Formulary. British Medical Association and Royal Pharmaceutical Society of Great Britain, London.

British National Formulary for Children. British Medical Association and Royal Pharmaceutical Society of Great Britain, London.

Deary IJ, Frier BM (1999). Glycaemic control in diabetes. *BMJ* **319**, 104–106.

Richter B, Neises G (2004). 'Human' insulin versus animal insulin in people with diabetes mellitus. *Cochrane Database of Systematic Reviews* **3**.

Driver and Vehicle Licensing Authority. *At a glance Guide to the current Medical Standards of Fitness to Drive*. Available at: http://www.dvla.gov.uk/medical/ataglance.aspx.

CHAPTER 11

Self-Management of Diabetes

Tim Holt[1] and Sudhesh Kumar[2]

[1]Nuffield Department of Primary Care Health Sciences, Oxford University, UK
[2]Warwick Medical School, University of Warwick; and WISDEM, University Hospital, Coventry, UK

OVERVIEW

- The emphasis of modern diabetes care is on self-management, which is appropriate for the majority of patients.
- People living with diabetes vary enormously in their individual needs and expectations.
- Patients and clinicians should work together to set priorities, define targets and overcome barriers to quality of life.

Introduction

The clinic consultation is a valuable, but very brief, window of opportunity for advice and reflection on progress towards treatment targets. New technologies have increased the availability of clinician advice to patients in ways not foreseen a generation ago. For the majority of the time, however, patients make their own hour-by-hour decisions about what to eat, how much insulin to take and how to adapt this to immediate needs, including exercise requirements. Clinicians need to encourage patients to learn self-management skills.

Important issues for the individual include:

- What should I eat?
- How should I self-monitor and how frequently?
- How can I interpret and act on the results of my blood tests to improve control?
- How can I exercise effectively and safely, to encourage weight loss and improve my health?

What should I eat?

By and large, people with diabetes should be encouraged to eat a similar healthy diet as that recommended to the general population. NICE recommends that people at high risk of (or with) CVD eat a cardioprotective diet in which total fat intake is 30% or less of total energy intake, saturated fats are 7% or less of total energy intake, intake of dietary cholesterol is less than 300 mg/day and,

where possible, saturated fats are replaced by mono-unsaturated and polyunsaturated fats. However, some patients are unclear about what this actually means in practice and some elements are of particular importance for people with diabetes (see Box 11.1).

The modern approach aims to induce sustainable lifestyle changes and avoids the term 'diabetic diet'. Most type 2 patients are either overweight or obese, and are likely to benefit from weight loss. Individuals differ in their preferences and responses to weight loss interventions but all are likely to need ongoing support to achieve sustained changes in eating habits and maintain their weight loss. For those who are overweight or obese, successful weight control is the most important objective.

Patients need to understand the different types of carbohydrate and the rate at which glucose is released into the blood stream as well as the appropriate amounts of carbohydrate foods to consume. This is reflected in the overall glycaemic load of the diet (the product of total carbohydrate x glycaemic index). However, any approach that achieves consistent weight loss is also likely to benefit glycaemic control and the need for medication. People with diabetes are at increased risk of CVD, so interventions to control dyslipidaemia (notably decreasing saturated fat and increasing dietary fibre) and hypertension (especially reductions in salt and increases in potassium intake), are also important.

Recommended approach to healthy eating for people with type 2 diabetes (Diabetes UK)

- *Eat regular meals.* Spacing meals evenly throughout the day will help control your appetite and blood glucose levels, especially if you are on twice-daily insulin.
- *Include starchy carbohydrates.* Carbohydrate (carbs) affects blood glucose levels, so be conscious of how much you eat, and opt for carbs that are more slowly absorbed. Try: pasta, basmati or easy-cook rice; granary, pumpernickel or rye bread; new potatoes, sweet potatoes and yams; oat-based cereals, such as porridge or natural muesli.
- *Cut the fat.* Eat less fat - particularly saturated fat. Try: unsaturated fats and oils, especially mono-unsaturated fats such as extra virgin olive oil and rapeseed oil, as these types of fat are better for

your heart; using skimmed or semi-skimmed milk and other low-fat dairy products; grilling, steaming or baking foods instead of frying.

- *Try to eat five a day.* Aim for at least five portions of fruit and/or vegetables every day to give your body the vitamins, minerals and fibre it needs. A portion is: 1 piece of fruit, like a banana or apple, 1 handful of grapes, 1 tablespoonful of dried fruit, 1 small glass of fruit juice or fruit smoothie, 3 heaped tablespoonful of vegetables.
- *Eat plenty of beans.* Beans, lentils and pulses are all low in fat, high in fibre and cheap to buy. They do not have a big impact on blood glucose, and may help to control blood fats such as cholesterol. Try kidney beans, chickpeas, green lentils, and even baked beans – hot in soups and casseroles, cold in salads, in baked falafel, bean burgers and low-fat hummus and dahls.
- *Eat more fish.* All types of fish are healthy, provided they are not coated in batter or fried, but oily fish such as mackerel, sardines, salmon and trout are particularly good for you. They are rich in omega-3 (polyunsaturated fat), which helps protect against heart disease. Aim to eat two portions of oily fish a week, ideally from a sustainable source.
- *Cut back on sugar.* This does not mean you need to eat a sugar-free diet. You can include some sugar in foods, including baked foods, in a healthy, balanced diet, provided you do not overdo it – just aim to have less of it. You can also use sweeteners as an alternative to sugar. Some easy ways to cut back on your sugar intake are: choosing sugar-free, no-added sugar or diet/light drinks; buying canned fruit in juice rather than syrup; reducing or cutting out sugar in tea and coffee. Remember, sugary drinks are an excellent treatment for hypos.
- *Reduce your salt.* Too much salt can raise your blood pressure, which increases your risk of heart disease and stroke. Reduce salt in your diet to 6 g or less a day. Try: Cutting back on processed foods, which account for 70% of our salt intake; flavouring foods with herbs and spices instead of salt.
- *Drink sensibly.* The recommended daily alcohol limit for women is 2-3 units, and 3-4 units for men.

Remember: 1 unit is a single measure (25ml) of spirits, ½ pint (284ml) of lager, beer or cider or a 175 ml glass of wine. Alcohol is high in calories so, to lose weight, consider cutting back. Never drink on an empty stomach, as alcohol can make hypos more likely to happen, if you are at risk of hypos.

- *Avoid diabetic foods.* These products offer no benefit to people with diabetes and may still affect your blood glucose levels. They contain as much fat and calories as ordinary versions, are expensive and can have a laxative effect.

Reducing glycaemic load

Glycaemic load is the product of net carbohydrate × glycaemic index (GI). The net carbohydrate is the total carbohydrate minus dietary fibre. The glycaemic index (GI) is a measure of the overall effect on blood glucose of an ingested carbohydrate source. Complex carbohydrate sources have a lower GI than simple sugars. Reducing glycaemic load is likely to benefit both weight and glycaemia, provided the person does not compensate by increasing fat intake, as this will increase weight and insulin resistance. Lists are available of the GIs of several hundred foods.

There is some evidence that low GI diets can assist in glycaemic control by smoothing blood glucose fluctuations and improving satiety, assisting in weight loss. Changing from bread and potatoes to pasta and Basmati rice as the main carbohydrate staples is likely to be beneficial for many patients, as it reduces glycaemic index and, therefore, glycaemic load (provided the total carbohydrate is the same).

However, the measurement of glycaemic index is problematic and foods may affect glycaemia inconsistently – depending, for instance, on the other foods consumed. Patients may develop misconceptions about the best food options and may exclude potentially healthy food rich in nutrients, such as root vegetables. Individual dietetic advice is beneficial to clarify these issues.

Modern nutritional management

The modern focus is on encouraging an interesting, varied diet with regular intake of complex carbohydrate (CHO). Even though such CHO is calorific, it is less so than an equivalent weight of fat, and it tends to satisfy the appetite more effectively as it will be absorbed over a longer period of time. Simple sugars should be kept to a minimum, but are not completely disallowed and they may, in small amounts, make the diet more appealing.

The challenge is to reduce calorie intake in a sustainable way. Referral to a dietician (see Box 11.2) is recommended for all patients at diagnosis.

A few additional points of advice may be helpful to supplement the 'healthy eating' message:

- Planning meals and, if necessary, including healthy snacks, is a vital skill to help people establish healthy eating habits.
- Fruit is recommended on a regular basis, but *fruit juice* is surprisingly high in carbohydrate and calories and should be limited to a maximum of 150ml a day.
- Patients sometimes take away with the 'healthy eating' message an assumption that drinks such as cola and lemonade are 'healthier' than their low-calorie equivalents, as they are less likely to contain artificial ingredients. In fact, such drinks are loaded with simple carbohydrate, and their exclusion may help very significantly in reducing calorie intake and blood sugar

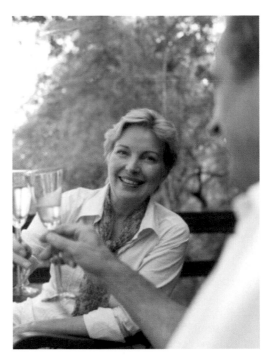

Figure 11.1 Alcohol should be taken only with awareness of the risks, which are higher in those with diabetes. Source: Digital image courtesy of the Getty's Open Content Program

levels. Some patients may have been self-treating the thirst of hyperglycaemia with these drinks prior to diagnosis. Low-calorie alternatives, containing no carbohydrate at all, are now widely available and generally safe (the exception is that people with phenylketonuria should avoid aspartame, which contains phenylalanine).

- Food should remain interesting. A simple piece of advice is to encourage patients to ensure their plate contains foods of several different colours (a 'rainbow' – see Chapter 21).
- Salad foods are available all the year round, and should not be viewed as exclusively a summer option.
- Although most foods can be taken at least 'occasionally', there is a danger that patients may consume a different 'occasional treat' item on each day of the week, believing (correctly, in a sense) that they have followed the advice. This may be one reason why a patient fails to lose weight.
- Processed foods including sauces often contain a lot of added salt, which manufacturers know will make them more likely to sell. The 6 g/day limit is on sodium *chloride* and this equates to 2.4 g of sodium, as salt is only 40% sodium. This is important, as manufacturers often give the content simply as sodium, which does not sound as high.
- Understanding appropriate portion sizes for food is important to help control calorie intake. The recommend serving size on the pack is a useful guide. Many people will benefit from weighing out a portion of foods such as pasta, rice or breakfast cereal that they consume regularly to help identify an appropriate portion.

Alcohol

Alcohol is not excluded in diabetes, and in moderation carries some cardiovascular benefits, but the following issues are very important:

- Many alcoholic drinks are highly calorific, partly because the alcohol itself is so, even when not combined with sweet ingredients.
- Sweet alcoholic drinks include sherries and liqueurs. These not only contain calories, but also sugar that is likely to raise blood glucose levels.
- The same applies to beers, even 'bitters', particularly the darker ones.
- Lagers, or dry wines in strict moderation, are therefore preferable.

- Intoxication with alcohol may impair an individual's ability to control their diabetes, for instance through their decision-making over carbohydrate intake and insulin doses.
- Alcohol may mask the symptoms of hypoglycaemia – the patient who is actually hypo may not receive assistance as it is clear they are intoxicated.
- Alcohol directly impairs the metabolic response to falling blood glucose.
- Alcohol interacts with sulphonylureas to increase the risk of hypoglycaemia.
- A combination of hypoglycaemia and alcohol intoxication puts the patient at risk of a seizure.

Individuals who wish to take alcohol need to be aware of all of these issues. A particularly dangerous situation is where insulin is taken at a social event, as well as alcohol, followed by delay in the arrival of the meal, leading to severe hypoglycaemia that is not recognised early enough by the intoxicated patient or his/her companions. It is often at social events where the individual loses control of meal arrangements (content and timing), and at the same events alcohol is frequently on offer (Figure 11.1).

Should I self-monitor?

In the UK, there is a national funding issue over self-monitoring, as testing strips are still quite expensive and are prescribed under the NHS. Most patients with diabetes get free prescriptions and the cost of this activity is, therefore, borne largely by the state. In countries without such a system, the cost is likely to fall on the individual, and any benefits may then add to health inequalities between socio-economic groups.

In selecting patients likely to benefit from self-monitoring, the following issues should be considered:

- **Treatment regimen**. Those taking insulin (particularly type 1 patients) are far more likely to benefit than patients treated with lifestyle measures alone or oral medication, for reasons discussed below. Type 1 patients are generally recommended to monitor at least twice a day. A Cochrane review (Malanda et al. 2012) concluded that in people with type 2 diabetes not treated with insulin, there was little if any effect of self-monitoring on HbA1c and no effect on patient satisfaction, general wellbeing or general health-related quality of life. However, those taking sulphonylureas or metaglinides may also be at risk of hypo and in many cases should be advised to self-monitor, particularly if they drive a car.
- **Symptom awareness**. Some patients are better than others at predicting their current blood glucose level without monitoring and may be able to predict whether it is likely to be rising, falling or static. Those who have lost hypoglycaemia awareness are particularly dependent on frequent monitoring. Others may tend to mistake normal symptoms (e.g. of hunger or anxiety) for hypoglycaemia.
- **The need for flexibility**. For some patients, flexibility in carbohydrate intake and exercise is required for their lifestyle, which might include frequent international travel, night shifts or unpredictable delays in mealtimes. Such influences should not be encouraged, as they are likely to be disruptive; however, if they are unavoidable, then frequent monitoring combined with appropriate adjustments may maintain stability. Patients driving for long distances and at any risk of hypoglycaemia should generally monitor before setting off and every 90–120 minutes during the journey. For patients wishing to fast during Ramadan, self-monitoring is often recommended during this period.
- **Response to abnormal results**. It is part of the personality of some patients to 'over-react' to abnormal results. Such individuals, unless they can 'retrain' this tendency, are at risk of 'tampering' (i.e. of worsening, rather than improving control as a result of the monitoring). It is sometimes possible to identify such a predisposition among the behaviour of a patient in other areas of their life.
- **Other psychological issues**. 'Learned helplessness' is a potential psychological effect of self-monitoring in the patient who has not been taught (or is unable to learn) to respond appropriately to self-monitored results. It is, in a sense, the *opposite* of self-efficacy. Unexpected fluctuations become perplexing and demoralising. This may reduce quality of life, and can easily result if self-monitoring is recommended with no training in responding behaviourally to the results.

Continuous glucose monitoring devices

Figures 11.2 and 11.3 represent profiles from a type 2 and a type 1 patient respectively, using a continuous glucose monitoring device taking subcutaneous glucose measurements every five minutes for 72 hours. A subcutaneous probe is inserted under the skin. Such devices are now available to allow patients and clinicians to explore underlying patterns in blood glucose profiles, but the technology is still quite expensive for routine use.

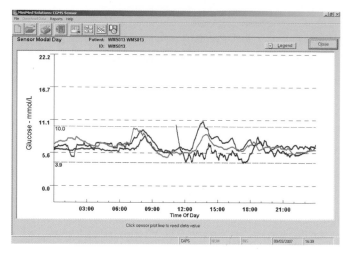

Figure 11.2 Profile from a patient with type 2 diabetes treated with metformin only. Fluctuations are relatively small and the fasting level is very similar on each of the days sampled. Source: Reproduced with permission of Medtronic.

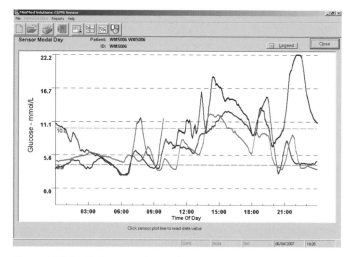

Figure 11.3 Profile from a patient with type 1 diabetes treated with an insulin pump. The HbA1c is similar to that in Figure 11.2. but the dynamical properties are clearly different. Source: Reproduced with permission of Medtronic.

How should I use my blood glucose results to improve control?

Chapter 3 discussed the now-established principle of patient autonomy, in succession to the more paternalistic approach of the past. This paternalism arose at a time when self-monitoring at home was not a practical proposition – the technology had simply not been invented. Patients depended much more on a doctor's advice to achieve glycaemic control, and might need admission to hospital to measure the diurnal profile over a period of days. This approach is still required in difficult cases, including the more brittle patterns seen in children.

Self-monitoring technology has changed this situation, as a patient can now easily build such a profile through regular

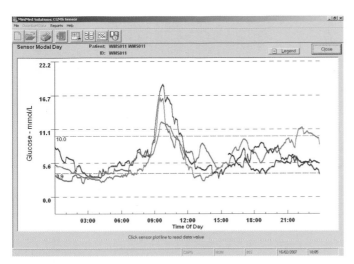

Figure 11.4 Increase in blood glucose after breakfast on each of the three monitoring days during a continuous glucose monitoring system (CGMS) recording. A self-monitoring schedule, involving measurements four times a day (before each meal and at bedtime), would have missed these excursions. Source: Reproduced with permission of Medtronic.

monitoring in the more natural environment of their usual daily activities (see Box 11.3).

Retrospective analysis

The traditional approach aims to identify patterns that are only evident when several days or more of data are gathered and examined in retrospect. This may improve understanding of the dynamic behaviour. Software is available to enable sharing of the data between patient and clinician via the internet (see Figure 11.5). However, there are several limitations of this approach.

First, the profile may be 'complete', but significant excursions may occur between monitoring (see Figure 11.4). Carbohydrate intake and insulin doses may be recorded much less consistently than the glucose data, and exercise is very difficult to quantify. Data may be uploaded to a personal computer to assist with

processing and statistical evaluation but, more often, the raw data are presented without any such tools. The human eye struggles to perceive patterns in numerical data, particularly when decimal places are used, which is why graphical displays may be very helpful.

Second, the assumption is often made that the profile has been gathered without the emerging results influencing the patient's behaviour, as it might if we were collecting it during a study on an animal or during a 'blinded' monitoring exercise. However, the patient's responses to the readings may be a powerful determinant of the dynamic behaviour. High fasting levels may arise through over-correction of nocturnal hypoglycaemia, for instance, but such details may not be recorded in the profile.

Despite these limitations, the following guidelines may help improve control based on retrospective analysis of the profile.

Advice based on the retrospective approach

Unless there is good reason to alter doses acutely (such as imminent hypoglycaemia or intercurrent illness), for most patients it is best to keep doses fairly stable (with less than 10% change) from day to day. Patterns of variation are more important than single random glucose values.

Examine the profile and attempt to identify consistent, *reproducible* peaks and troughs.

To increase blood glucose in the troughs
- Eat more carbohydrate at, or before, the times when blood glucose values are at their lowest – usually at mid-morning and at bed-time.
- Reduce the dose of insulin before the trough.
- Consider changing a short-acting insulin to a rapid-acting insulin analogue to avoid pre meal hypoglycaemia.

To decrease blood glucose in the peaks
- Reduce carbohydrate intake at the meals that precede the peaks.
- Increase the dose of insulin before the peak.

These adjustments should be made with an awareness of the duration of action of the various types of insulin (see Chapter 9).

To decrease fasting hyperglycaemia
- Increase the evening intermediate- or long-acting insulin.
- If this causes nocturnal hypoglycaemia, consider splitting the pre-dinner insulin into two parts, with the short- or rapid-acting insulin before dinner and the longer-acting insulin at bedtime. Alternatively, if the patient is taking an intermediate-acting insulin in the evening, consider changing to a long-acting insulin analogue such as detemir or glargine.

To reduce nocturnal hypoglycaemia
- Reduce the dose of the evening intermediate-acting insulin or long-acting insulin analogue.
- Advise the patient to take carbohydrate at bedtime. This is particularly important if the bedtime blood glucose level is < 6.0 mmol/l.

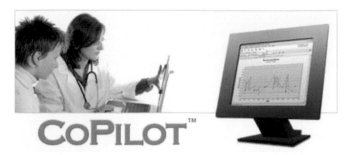

Figure 11.5 The *CoPilot* program for assisting in management of diabetes. Source: Reproduced with kind permission from Abbott Laboratories Limited.

- Consider changing evening intermediate-acting insulin to a long-acting insulin analogue to avoid nocturnal 'peaking' of insulin levels.

Software programs have been designed to assist in dose adjustment to optimise insulin regimens. These include the *CoPilot* system (see Figure 11.5).

The prospective approach

In the past, the retrospective approach was promoted as the only appropriate technique, but it may seem like 'driving a car by looking through the rear mirror', to quote one patient. This is a particular problem if lifestyles require flexibility, and immediate needs are inconsistent from one day to the next. To continue the metaphor, patients are likely to want to use the front windscreen *prospectively*, as well as the rear mirror retrospectively, but there are dangers if the patient is not sufficiently skilled at this.

Some of the problems with prospective responses to blood glucose results include:

- **'Chasing the tail'**. Displacement of the glucose level is detected, but the response is to over-correct, resulting in displacement in the opposite direction. This may again lead to over-correction, repeating the cycle, and so on.
- **Overlap of insulin doses**. Self-monitoring may occur before the most recent insulin dose has taken full effect, so that a high blood glucose level is treated with an unnecessary corrective dose, when restoration of a normal level would have occurred without any interference.
- **Inappropriate adjustment of long-acting insulin**. In another common scenario, the patient detects a raised measurement prior to the daily long-acting insulin dose, and increases the long-acting dose accordingly. This action is delayed, and then overlaps with other insulin doses hours later or the following day.
- **Inappropriate response to a non-significant fluctuation in the glucose level**. As Figure 11.3 demonstrates, glucose levels may fluctuate quite widely over a period of an hour or two, and some of this fluctuation represents dynamic 'noise' that should be ignored rather than used as a basis for prospective action. Impulsive responses to such noise will worsen control.

These problems are typical of the 'tampering' phenomenon, in which self-monitoring results in deterioration rather than improvement in control, justifying past caution over this prospective approach. However, the modern patient is likely to want to develop prospective control skills to provide flexibility (Figure 11.6). The DAFNE approach (Box 11.4) involves an individually tailored

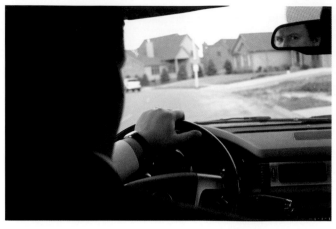

Figure 11.6 The retrospective and prospective approaches should, ideally, complement each other. After all, no good driver attempts to control the vehicle without using both the windscreen and the rear mirrors.

Box 11.4 **DAFNE**

DAFNE ('Dose Adjustment For Normal Eating') is a five-day training programme for adults with type 1 diabetes, and involves accurate carbohydrate counting and adjustment of insulin doses, according to need. It is suitable for well-motivated patients who have been diagnosed for at least six months, and who are prepared to monitor 4–6 times a day and inject insulin frequently. It is based on the idea that tailoring insulin doses to the person's usual diet (which is, in principle, unrestricted) is the best way of achieving glycaemic control without increased hypoglycaemia. It has been shown in a randomised controlled trial to improve HbA1c levels (as well as quality of life scores) without increasing the frequency of severe hypoglycaemia. It is not known whether long-term metabolic outcomes are affected by the dietary freedom, but short-term cardiovascular risk factors were unaffected.

The details of the DAFNE approach are not widely available, as it is important that patients using this technique are properly trained by attending the five-day course. For the reference to the DAFNE trial report, see Chapter 3. For details on how to apply or refer, see: www.dafne.uk.com

---

algorithm for dose adjustment, combined with accurate carbohydrate counting. There is no dietary restriction, and insulin doses are adapted to carbohydrate intake choices. It is the only evidenced-based programme currently on offer for type 1 patients wishing to adjust doses flexibly. An adapted programme for the 11–16 year age group is under development.

Self-monitoring techniques

There is now a wide variety of self-monitoring systems available. It is preferable for the whole health care team to be familiar with the same device or a small number of alternatives.

While the devices are not themselves prescribable in the UK, manufacturers will usually supply them free of charge to diabetes teams (e.g. general practices or hospital diabetes centres) to distribute to patients. The testing strips can then be prescribed.

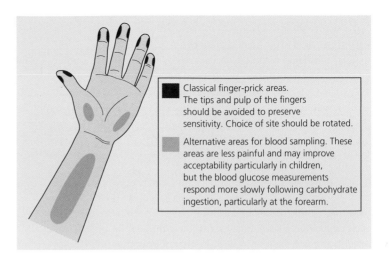

Figure 11.7 Sites on the hand suitable for blood sampling.

The monitors must be user-friendly in a range of environments, and the best options will provide the following features:

- Small, compact, and easily carried in clothing or a handbag.
- Only require a small amount of blood for a measurement.
- Beep to confirm that sufficient blood has been applied, but not so loudly that monitoring cannot be done discreetly.
- Give an accurate reading in a short time frame (e.g. 12 seconds).
- Do not require blood to be 'wiped off' the end of the strip.
- Have a luminescent screen, and so usable in the dark.
- Use testing strips that can be disposed of by flushing away.
- Preferably include the option of testing for blood ketones.
- Have a memory for recall of past results.
- Increasingly, patients will want to upload results to a personal computer for retrospective analysis, a feature available with some, but not all, devices.
- Some monitors will advise type 1 patients on the insulin dose required, based on current blood glucose measurement, estimated carbohydrate in the forthcoming meal, and the patient's usual carbohydrate to insulin ratio at that time of day.

Blood may be taken from the distal edges of the fingers (the central pulp of the fingers should be avoided, to preserve nerve ending function in the long run), from the forearms (less pain-sensitive), from the thenar or hypothenar eminences (see Figure 11.7), or from the earlobes (which are usually very vascular and bleed easily, even when other sites do not).

Ideal frequency of self-monitoring

The expected benefits and frequency of self-monitoring should be agreed between patient and clinician before starting. Patients on insulin, whose diabetes is intensively (and 'prospectively') managed, will need to monitor 4–6 times per day to gain maximum benefit, particularly when flexibility is required. Other patients, including those with type 2 diabetes whose carbohydrate intake is relatively constant in quantity and timing, will require readings less often, provided hypoglycaemia awareness is intact.

For patients who are not taking drugs producing risk of hypo (insulin, sulphonylureas, glinides), but in whom it has been decided that monitoring is beneficial, a measurement taken twice a week may be appropriate, increased during illness. Those taking oral medication (and certainly those taking insulin) may benefit from monitoring

Box 11.5 **Sick Day Rules**

Glycaemic control may become very difficult during intercurrent illness, particularly when vomiting occurs. The basic principles are to monitor frequently (every 2–4 hours), to not stop insulin (as more than the usual dose is typically needed), to titrate insulin doses to blood glucose results, and to maintain a regular intake of easily digested simple carbohydrate. If this is not possible, admission to hospital is needed. Regular testing of the urine or blood for ketones during the illness is useful to detect the onset of ketoacidosis, which requires prompt treatment with intravenous fluids and insulin.

In addition to blood glucose control during acute illnesses, there is a need to omit certain medications until fully recovered. These include, in particular, angiotensin-converting enzyme inhibitors (or angiotensin 2 receptor blockers) which, despite long term reno-protective effects, can cause acute kidney injury (AKI) in the acutely ill or dehydrated patient. Diuretics should also be omitted if fluid volume is depleted. Metformin can rarely cause lactic acidosis, and this risk is much higher during acute illness and dehydration.

before driving – a policy recommended by the Driving and Vehicle Licensing Authority. Insulin users should monitor before setting off, and every 90–120 minutes during the journey. Ramadan is a situation when individuals who do not usually monitor may benefit from doing so. The frequency of self-monitoring should be increased at times of sickness, particularly for type 1 patients (Box 11.5).

New technologies

The past 15 years have seen a rapid development of technologies to assist patients in self-management. These include computer-assisted self-management programmes and flow sheets, telemedicine options, internet-based educational software and automated telephone products. In a systematic review in 2006, Jackson and colleagues found that, as well as improvements in HbA1c reported in most studies, IT-based interventions improved health care utilisation, behaviours, attitudes, knowledge and skills. However, ethnic minorities are not well-represented in the research literature and, unless the problem of access is addressed, the development of such technologies is likely to widen, rather than reduce, health inequalities.

Maintaining an active lifestyle

Physical activity and diabetes

Regular moderate aerobic physical activity for at least 30 minutes on five days of the week, recommended for the whole population, is particularly valuable in those with diabetes. Generally speaking, the activity should be sufficient to make the person breathless and raise the heart rate. This activity should:

- increase the chances of sustained weight loss;
- improve the lipid profile;
- reduce blood pressure.

It also increases insulin sensitivity and can improve glycaemic control, provided appropriate account is taken for the exercise in adjusting insulin doses and carbohydrate intake. Increasing the exercise beyond a moderate level is likely to result in little further benefit, and may be risky. The risks are not only those of hypoglycaemia (particularly in insulin-treated patients), but also of actual physical injury. A sprained ankle is easily acquired and may preclude exercise for several weeks.

For some patients, obesity and associated arthritis or other physical problems may make exercise difficult or impossible. Advice and guidance is now widely available through personal trainers, but such people must be adequately trained themselves. Swimming is usually a safe and effective form of exercise, as is brisk walking. For those who cannot manage this, any amount of physical activity, however small, is better than nothing, and some people may be able to increase their activity significantly simply by rearranging their work environment. Using a toilet on a different floor, avoiding using a lift, walking to visit others in different office rooms, rather than telephoning, and other simple changes to everyday habits may be very beneficial.

Summary

The emphasis of diabetes care is on self-management, but the availability of medical expertise is as important as ever. Patients need to be taught a range of skills in order to take control and 'ownership' of their condition. These include advice on nutritional management and exercise to achieve sustained weight loss and improved cardiovascular risk, and training in managing blood glucose levels through self-monitoring where appropriate. Through these measures, the patient can work together with the health care team to develop the confidence and self-efficacy needed to overcome the day-to-day challenges of diabetes.

Further reading and references

Malanda UL, Welschen LMC, Riphagen II, *et al.* (2012). Self-monitoring of blood glucose in patients with type 2 diabetes mellitus who are not using insulin (Review). Cochrane Database Syst Rev: 1: CD005060.

Jackson CL, Bolen S, Brancati FL, *et al.* (2006). A Systematic Review of Interactive Computer-assisted Technology in Diabetes Care. *Journal of General Internal Medicine* **21**,105–110.

Connor H, Annan F, Bunn E, Frost G, McGough N, Sarwar T, Thomas B; Nutrition Subcommittee of the Diabetes Care Advisory Committee of Diabetes UK (2003). The implementation of nutritional advice for people with diabetes. *Diabetic Medicine* **20**, 786–807.

Department of Health (2001). The expert patient: a new approach to chronic disease management for the twenty-first century. London: Department of Health. www.ohn.gov.uk/ohn/people/expert

Tattersall R (2002). The expert patient: A new approach to chronic disease management for the twenty-first century. *Clinical Medicine* **2**, 227–229.

CHAPTER 12

Surveillance for Complications

Tim Holt[1] and Sudhesh Kumar[2]

[1]Nuffield Department of Primary Care Health Sciences, Oxford University, UK
[2]Warwick Medical School, University of Warwick; and WISDEM, University Hospital, Coventry, UK

OVERVIEW

- Early detection of complications requires a systematic surveillance programme involving regular review, examination and blood monitoring.

- Complications particularly amenable to early detection include retinopathy, microalbuminuria and foot ulceration risk.

- Surveillance also provides opportunities for review of control of the key cardiovascular risk factors: glycaemia, blood pressure and lipids.

- Regular contact facilitates discussion on factors affecting quality of life including mood, hypoglycaemia, erectile dysfunction and driving safety.

Introduction

Once the diagnosis of diabetes is confirmed, the patient should be entered into a structured programme of surveillance and follow-up. The purpose of surveillance is twofold: to identify the development of complications as early as possible; and to address factors that can be treated to prevent or delay their onset. The importance of this programme must be clearly explained as part of the initial patient education, emphasising its benefits and evidence base.

Structure of a basic surveillance programme

This chapter describes the techniques used to conduct diabetes surveillance (Box 12.1). Treatments and targets are discussed elsewhere in the book. Most of the surveillance measures required should be conducted at least annually. As discussed in Chapter 19, a regular habit of annual review is important, both to improve concordance and to ensure that the process is completed. If some of the measures are taken opportunistically, outside the annual review appointments, then this may reduce the effectiveness of the programme as the patient may be less inclined to attend for the remaining checks. However, blood pressure, glycaemic control and monitoring of renal function usually need to be carried out more frequently, outside of the annual reviews.

Weight and body mass index

Weight is a good index of the success of lifestyle change. Ninety percent of patients with type 2 diabetes are overweight or obese at diagnosis and benefit from weight reduction, particularly when this is associated with increased physical activity. Abdominal obesity carries a particularly raised risk of cardiovascular disease, so waist measurement is also useful to monitor success in reducing this risk factor. The patient should usually be weighed with coat and shoes off, but otherwise clothed, on regularly calibrated scales, and preferably the same scales each time (Figure 12.1).

Blood pressure measurement

Blood pressure should be taken with the patient sitting down and after a few minutes rest, with the cuff at the same level as the heart and the elbow very slightly flexed (Figure 12.2). An appropriately sized cuff is important, as too small a cuff will give falsely raised readings. Initially, it is worth checking the blood pressure in both arms and, if there is consistent difference then the arm with the highest pressure should be used in future for monitoring. It is also useful to measure the sitting and standing blood pressure, and this should be done annually, particularly in elderly patients.

A fall of greater than 20 mm Hg after standing may be a sign of autonomic neuropathy (see Chapter 16). If such a fall is associated with postural hypotension symptoms, this will affect blood pressure management and may be a contraindication to drug therapy. Alternatively, it may be associated with one of the drugs currently used to reduce blood pressure, in which case it may resolve when this drug is stopped or changed to an alternative. Beta blockers, thiazide diuretics and alpha blockers are particularly likely to cause postural hypotension.

ABC of Diabetes, Seventh Edition. Tim Holt and Sudhesh Kumar.
© 2015 John Wiley & Sons, Ltd. Published 2015 by John Wiley & Sons, Ltd.

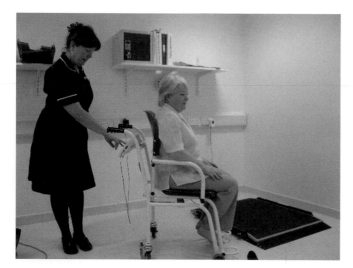

Figure 12.1 Weight measurement at the University Hospital, Coventry. The black mat on the floor in the background is a device for measuring very heavy patients over 200 kg.

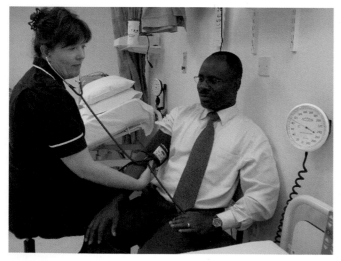

Figure 12.2 Blood pressure measurement.

Cholesterol and lipids

Patients should ideally have a fasting lipid profile measured annually, to include total serum cholesterol, HDL, LDL and fasting triglycerides. The majority of patients should be prescribed a lipid-lowering agent (see Chapter 6), irrespective of their baseline serum cholesterol.

It will usually, therefore, be advisable to check the liver function tests on at least an annual basis.

Glycosylated haemoglobin (HbA1c)

HbA1c is a reflection of average blood glucose values over the previous 2–3 months. Measurement should be made every six months, or at the very least annually. There is little point in repeating the measurement earlier than two months following a change in therapy, as it takes this long to change in response to red blood cell turnover. Other means of gauging control (including self-monitored blood glucose levels and symptoms of hypoglycaemia) may be used in the meantime to guide decisions on treatment.

Estimated glomerular filtration rate (e-GFR)

While at best an approximation, this marker is a much more adequate index of renal function than serum creatinine, as it takes account of age, sex and ethnicity. In the UK, the e-GFR can be requested on a blood sample at the same time as urea, electrolytes and creatinine, and is calculated automatically by the laboratory using the MDRD formula (although the adjustment for ethnicity is not included). The e-GFR should be measured at least annually, and more frequently in patients whose renal function is reduced or at risk of declining, in those taking medication that can affect renal function, such as diuretics, non-steroidal anti-inflammatory drugs or ACE inhibitors, and those taking drugs that are contraindicated if renal function is poor (such as metformin). Such decisions are much more securely based on e-GFR than on serum creatinine measurements.

More than one e-GFR measurement is required to confirm renal impairment, and unexpectedly low values should be followed up by repeated measurements to confirm (as well as to exclude progressive decline), as levels may be artificially reduced in the short term by dehydration, recent changes in medication or other factors. To maximise the validity of an e-GFR measurement, the patient should avoid ingesting meat for 12 hours before the blood sampling.

Foot examination

All patients with diabetes should have a thorough foot examination at least annually and, in those with signs of complications or 'at-risk' features, this frequency should be increased. The examination should include, as a minimum, the following:

- **Inspection of the general health of the feet**. Signs of deformity, hair loss, loss of skin integrity, loss of sweating, swelling of joints, callosities, nail health, fungal infection between the toes. Deformity or swelling may suggest an underlying Charcot's neuroarthropathy (see Chapter 15). Callosities suggest abnormal distribution of weight over the sole, which may indicate peripheral neuropathy.
- **Assessment of vascular sufficiency**. Temperature of the skin, detection of dorsalis pedis and posterior tibial pulses, capillary return at the toes. A Doppler device (Figure 12.3) may assist in assessing vascular sufficiency, particularly when used in experienced hands to measure ankle brachial pressure index. However, if the pedal pulses cannot be detected manually, then the arterial supply should be considered abnormal.

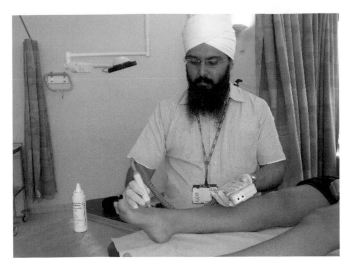

Figure 12.3 Identifying pedal pulses using a Doppler device at the University Hospital, Coventry. Source: Photograph courtesy of Mr G Deogan.

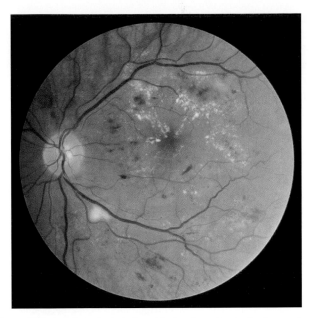

Figure 12.5 A digital retinal photograph showing extensive background and macular changes. Source: Photograph courtesy of Dr Paul O'Hare.

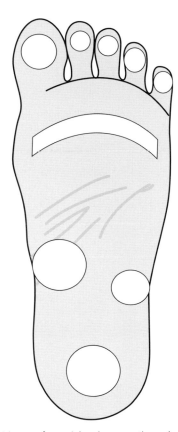

Figure 12.4 At-risk areas for peripheral neuropathy and neuropathic ulceration.

- **Assessment of neurological integrity**. Light touch sensation using a 10 g nylon microfibre device at all of the 'at-risk' areas (see Chapter 15, Figure 15.5) and vibration sense at the great toe and ankle; Achilles tendon reflex (Figure 12.4).

Advice and treatment of foot complications is covered in Chapter 15.

Digital retinal photography

Traditional fundoscopic examination, even in experienced hands and following dilatation of the pupils, is not an adequate means of excluding early retinopathy. The gold standard technique is digital retinal photography of both eyes following dilatation, and examination of the images by an experienced professional who analyses such images regularly (Figure 12.5). Dilatation should be achieved using a short-acting topical mydriatic such as tropicamide 0.5%. Retinopathy is present at the time of diagnosis in a proportion of type 2 patients (37% in the UKPDS study), and newly diagnosed individuals should not be left to wait 12 months before the annual screen is organised.

Urinary microalbumin screening

Dipstix are available for the detection of microalbumin but, for accurate quantification, a laboratory will measure the albumin: creatinine ratio. This is abnormal if > 2.5 for men and > 3.5 for women. A positive finding should be followed up with a second sample, as spurious positive results may occur, particularly if infection is present. If unconfirmed on a second sample, then a third should be arranged, and two out of three positive is considered conclusive. Angiotensin-converting enzyme inhibitors (ACEI) and tight control of blood pressure in patients with urinary microalbumin are extremely beneficial (see Chapter 13).

Depression screening

As with many long-term health problems, patients with diabetes are at significantly higher risk of depression, and symptoms may not be reported. Active questioning to screen for depressive symptoms could be part of an annual diabetes review. Positive indications of an underlying depression should be followed by a formal assessment, using a validated instrument such as the PHQ-9 (see Chapter 17).

Other issues

Other issues that need to be addressed on a regular basis include:

- **Erectile dysfunction**. Unless clearly inappropriate, a question about erectile dysfunction should be included in an annual review to male patients. This problem is common and treatable, but may go unreported because of embarrassment. If medication is required (e.g. Sildenafil), this should be placed in the 'Repeats' screen, along with other medication, unless there is a reason not to.
- **Driving safety**. The annual review is a good opportunity to discuss the patient's safety to drive a vehicle if appropriate. The regulations change from time to time and should be kept under review. The current rules are discussed separately in Chapter 10.
- **A holistic perspective**. It is easy to become fixated on 'box-ticking' when conducting surveillance reviews. Box-ticking is, in fact, extremely important if an assessment is to be comprehensive, and screen templates may facilitate this process. However, an assessment should also include some protected time for the 'free-text' issues that are important for quality of life. This is, after all, one of the major goals of diabetes management. These aspects are not as easily quantified or measured, but they are valued by patients. Relationship issues, educational progress, family support, work stress and other anxieties, and future life plans may all come to light to a receptive ear in a supportive environment. Spending time on these will build the clinician-patient relationship, and reap benefits in future when difficult management decisions need to be shared.

Summary

Surveillance for complications is a major component of diabetes care, and should take the form of regular reviews (at least annually), with protected time for a comprehensive assessment of the patient's needs. It cannot be managed by a single health care professional, but requires a teamwork approach using a shared care protocol, adapted to locally available resources and understood by all involved. This protocol should, where possible, be discussed with the patient to facilitate the early detection and treatment of complications. Routine surveillance should also include an exploration of the psycho-social issues that affect quality of life but which may not otherwise be reported.

Further reading

Driving and Vehicle Licensing Authority. *'At a Glance' Guide to Medical Standards of Fitness to Drive*. www.dvla.gov.uk/medical/ataglance.aspx

National Institute for Health and Clinical Excellence. Clinical Guideline 87. *Diabetes type 2 (update)*.

CHAPTER 13

Kidney Disease in Diabetes

Tim Holt[1] and Sudhesh Kumar[2]

[1]Nuffield Department of Primary Care Health Sciences, Oxford University, UK
[2]Warwick Medical School, University of Warwick; and WISDEM, University Hospital, Coventry, UK

OVERVIEW

- Nephropathy may already be established at presentation in type 2 patients and is a common long-term complication for those with type 1 diabetes.

- An increasing proportion of patients are living long enough to develop end stage renal failure, requiring expansion of renal replacement services.

- Progression of renal impairment is reduced through control of blood pressure, glycaemia and lipids, and angiotensin-converting enzyme inhibition.

- Angiotensin-converting enzyme inhibitors should be offered to all patients with any degree of albuminuria, unless contraindicated.

- Monitoring of renal function is an important task for primary care, and thresholds for referral to secondary care should be locally agreed and widely understood.

- Renal impairment affects other aspects of diabetes management, including choice of drugs and dosages.

Introduction

Despite improvements in early detection, prevention and treatment, diabetic nephropathy is still a major cause of mortality and morbidity. At 25 years from diagnosis of diabetes, around one-third of type 1 patients and a fifth of those with type 2 have end stage renal failure, although these figures are improving. The development of proteinuria is usually the first indication. Worsening renal function makes associated hypertension more difficult to control, leading to more generalised vascular disease and further renal damage. Untreated, renal function may deteriorate to the point of dialysis dependence, typically over a period of years.

Looking on the brighter side, urinalysis detects, at an early stage, a problem whose natural history can now be modified and, where this is not possible or is unsuccessful, adequate quality of life can usually be maintained through dialysis or transplantation. Mortality rates in dialysis and transplant patients are falling. Urinary albumin can now be detected at concentrations lower than are possible through conventional urinalysis. As discussed below, this 'microalbumin' signals the need for active measures to control risk factors and prevent further progression.

Epidemiology

Diabetic nephropathy is the most common specific primary renal diagnosis in patients entering UK programmes for renal replacement therapy (RRT), accounting for around 26.1% of cases reported in 2013 (Rao et al, 2013). The ratio of men to women is 1.6, due to accompanying renovascular disease, which is commoner in men. The prevalence in the population is increasing, reflecting the rising prevalence of diabetes, improved survival and treatment and a rise in referral rates for RRT, particularly in the type 2 population, with better access to dialysis units.

Van Dijk and colleagues describe the variation across different European centres (Van Dijk *et al.* 2005). Their figures show a steady rise in incidence of RRT, particularly among type 2 patients, where an increase of nearly 12% per year was observed (Figure 13.1). In the older age groups, the ratio of men to women increased during this decade. Improved mortality rates from cardiovascular disease may partly explain this trend. Although survival rates for dialysis patients are generally improving, mortality among those with diabetic nephropathy is still higher than in those with other causes of renal disease, partly due to co-morbidity, including cardiovascular disease.

The cyclical nature of causation in diabetic nephropathy (Boxes 13.1 and 13.2) makes it extremely worthwhile as a preventive endeavour, because the benefits (e.g. of blood pressure control) feed back on themselves in the long run.

Clinical presentation

Type 1 patients rarely develop signs of nephropathy prior to five years following diagnosis of diabetes. They typically have normal blood pressure and renal function at presentation. Type 2 patients often have had diabetes for several years before diagnosis, and a

ABC of Diabetes, Seventh Edition. Tim Holt and Sudhesh Kumar.
© 2015 John Wiley & Sons, Ltd. Published 2015 by John Wiley & Sons, Ltd.

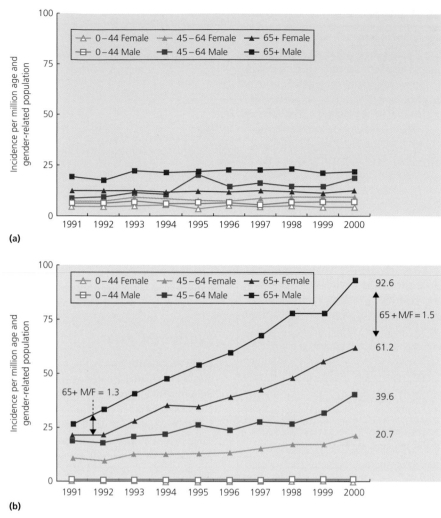

(a)

(b)

Figure 13.1 Incidence of renal replacement therapy (RRT) is relatively stable for type 1 patients **(a)** compared with type 2 populations **(b)**, where needs are escalating, particularly in older men. Source: Van Dijk *et al.* (2005). Reproduced with permission of Nature Publishing Group.

Box 13.1 **Breaking the Cycle**

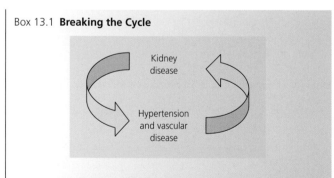

Pathological mechanisms in diabetic nephropathy are complex, and involve genetic factors as well as glycaemia, lipids, smoking and blood pressure. Microvascular and macrovascular factors conspire in the progression of this complication, a cycle reinforced by secondary hypertension.

Box 13.2 **Factors Promoting the Development and Progression of Nephropathy**

- Blood pressure.
- Poor glycaemic control.
- Dyslipidaemia.
- Smoking.
- High protein intake.
- Small kidneys.
- Genetic factors.

The stages of diabetic nephropathy (Table 13.1)
Decline in glomerular filtration rate (GFR)

The estimated GFR is a measure of creatinine clearance, and it progressively declines in patients with established diabetic nephropathy. However, as Table 13.1 indicates, prior to this decline the GFR may, in fact, be high. This generally applies at the stage of microalbuminuria (stage II) but also at the earlier stage I, which is not associated with any other abnormal investigation findings. This asymptomatic 'hyperfiltration' phase may or may not progress to the later stages, depending on how successfully

proportion have established nephropathy from the start. Many have co-existing hypertension and may be already at the stage of impaired renal function. Diabetic nephropathy can affect any patient, but is commoner in those of Afro-Caribbean and South Asian ethnicities.

Table 13.1 Stages of progression of diabetic nephropathy.

	Normal (I)	Incipient (II)	Persistent (III)	Clinical (IV)	End stage (V)
Albuminuria (mg/24 hours)	<20	20–300 (microalbuminuria)	≥300 (up to 15 g/day)	≥300 (up to 15 g/day)	≥300 (can fall)
Glomerular filtration rate (ml/min)	High/normal hyperfiltration	Normal/high	Normal or decreased	Decreased	Greatly decreased
Serum creatinine (μmol/l)	Normal 60–100	Normal 60–120	High normal 80–120	High 120–400	Very high > 400
Blood pressure (mm Hg)	Normal	Slightly increased	Increased	Increased	Increased
Clinical signs	None	None	Anaemia ± oedema, increased blood pressure, may be none	Anaemia ± oedema, increased blood pressure, may be none	Anaemia ± oedema, increased blood pressure, uraemic symptoms

Box 13.3 **Signs and Symptoms of Uraemia**

Malaise	**Nocturia**
Pallor	Dyspnoea
Hiccoughs	Oedema
Nausea	Confusion
Pruritis	Pericarditis

Table 13.2 Diagnostic definitions of microalbuminuria and proteinuria. An albumin creatinine ratio of 30 mg/mmol is approximately equivalent to a protein creatinine ratio of 50 mg/mmol.

	Urinary albumin concentration (mg/l)	Albumin: creatinine ratio	24-hour albumin excretion (mg/24 hr)
Normal	<20	<2.5 (men) <3.5 (women)	<30
Microalbuminuria	20–200	>2.5 (men) >3.5 (women)	30–300
Proteinuria	>200	>30	>300

Box 13.4 **Abrupt Onset of Proteinuria is Never Due to Diabetes**

Patients not following the typical pattern of presentation may have another cause of renal disease that might benefit from other types of treatment. Other causes are more likely to affect type 2 patients, as they tend to be commoner with increasing age.

blood pressure and other factors are controlled. Stage I individuals are not readily identifiable in clinical practice, but this should encourage clinicians to offer tight control of these risk factors to everyone with diabetes, all of whom are potentially at risk of nephropathy.

How will the patient feel?

The early stages of nephropathy are asymptomatic, which is one reason why screening is so important. Gradually, blood pressure may become more difficult to control, normocytic anaemia occurs, peripheral oedema may be evident, and the malaise and nausea of uraemia develop (Box 13.3). As renal function declines further, the symptoms related to uraemia and anaemia become progressively worse and, at this stage, the patient is entering an 'end stage' where the need for dialysis is impending.

Microalbuminuria

Renal damage is typically gradual and progressive, so the earlier it is detected, the better. Before the onset of proteinuria (in which albumin is detectable at a concentration of > 200 mg/l), milder degrees may be present that will be missed by conventional urinalysis. Detection of protein in the urine is more meaningful if it is measured as a ratio of urinary albumin to creatinine concentrations, or as a 24-hour excretion rate.

Microalbuminuria is defined as an albumin excretion rate of 30-300 mg/24 hours, or an albumin : creatinine ratio of > 2.5 mg/mmol/l (for men) and > 3.5 mg/mmol/l (for women) (Table 13.2). Stix are now available that can detect both microalbumin and creatinine to estimate this ratio. The first morning sample after rising is preferable to samples taken later in the day. Regular urinalysis for microalbumin should be part of routine surveillance in diabetes, but a positive finding must be repeated to confirm, and infection excluded as well. A sample should then be sent to the laboratory to measure the ratio more accurately or, alternatively, a 24-hour urine collection for albumin can be arranged.

Investigation of suspected nephropathy

Nephropathy is a well-recognised and not uncommon complication in diabetes, usually starting with albuminuria that progresses over time. However, other causes of kidney disease might affect someone with diabetes, and there are many potential causes of proteinuria. Therefore, the initial question is whether the diagnosis can be made based on the clinical presentation, or whether further investigations, including renal biopsy, are justified.

Patients with diabetes who develop microalbumin, and who are detected through routine surveillance, will not need invasive investigations at this stage. They should have a midstream specimen of urine (MSU) taken to exclude infection and, provided this is sterile and acellular, it is safe to continue follow-up on the assumption that they have stage II (incipient) nephropathy (see Table 13.1).

Those with actual proteinuria (detectable on conventional urinalysis suggesting a urinary albumin concentration > 200 mg/l) should similarly have infection, pyuria and haematuria excluded through MSU. It may be worth measuring albumin excretion through a 24-hour urine collection, to provide a baseline for future progression. Such patients should also have an ultrasound examination of the renal tract, to support the clinical examination in excluding unexpected pathology such as a tumour. For those with renal impairment, ultrasound also helps to exclude obstructive causes, particularly in men, who may have prostatic enlargement, or in either sex as a result of autonomic neuropathy causing chronic urinary retention (Box 13.4).

A blood test for C-reactive protein and antinuclear factor is worthwhile in patients with proteinuria. Routine biochemistry should reveal normal serum albumin levels. A patient with low albumin levels and oedema (nephrotic syndrome) is likely to have a different cause for their proteinuria (see Box 13.4). If the cause is diabetic nephropathy, at the point where proteinuria becomes detectable on conventional stix, it is likely that the e-GFR will be at least borderline, if not actually abnormal.

Patients with proteinuria due to diabetic nephropathy usually also have retinopathy. If this is not present, then other causes of renal disease need to be considered (Box 13.5).

Anaemia occurs relatively early in diabetic nephropathy, compared with other causes of kidney disease, so it is not unusual for this anaemia to be symptomatic at the point where the urea and creatinine are not particularly high.

Patients with renal artery stenosis may be identified if a decline in renal function (sometimes dramatic) occurs after commencing ACE inhibitors. A vascular bruit may be evident on auscultating the abdomen. Such patients should be referred for imaging of the renal arteries, and may benefit from interventions to improve renovascular function, including angioplasty.

Histological features of diabetic nephropathy

Renal biopsy

Renal biopsy is carried out via a posterior approach through the lumbar musculature, under local anaesthetic, and guided by ultrasound. In preparation, patients should have clotting function and platelet count checked, and should be fasted for six hours. Macroscopic haematuria frequently occurs after this procedure and is almost always self-limiting.

Histology

The typical histological signs of diabetic nephropathy are diabetic glomerulosclerosis with mesangial expansion and thickening of the basement membrane. The classical features evident in the later stages are Kimmelstiel-Wilson nodules, associated with hyalinisation of the efferent and afferent arterioles (Figure 13.2).

Primary prevention

Diabetic nephropathy is essentially a microvascular complication but, as indicated above, it may also trigger macrovascular processes that promote its further progression. This 'vicious cycle' should

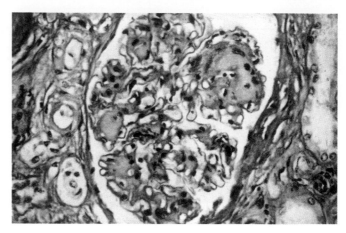

Figure 13.2 Diabetic glomerulosclerosis with Kimmelstiel-Wilson nodules.

encourage not only early intervention, but also prevention if possible. The most effective means of achieving this are through:
- Glycaemic control.
- Blood pressure control.
- Smoking cessation.

These should be offered to all patients with diabetes, but treatment targets should be tightened when the early stages of nephropathy develop. In patients with no current signs of nephropathy, targets need to be balanced against other issues, including quality of life and risks of over-treatment. This particularly applies to elderly patients and those whose life-expectancy is already limited.

Treatment of diabetic nephropathy

The patient with established nephropathy is not only at risk of end stage renal failure, but also of cardiovascular complications, including myocardial infarction. A high proportion of patients with proteinuria have co-existing coronary artery disease, which may be asymptomatic. It is also likely that other microvascular disease is present, and almost all have co-existing retinopathy.

Secondary prevention

The mainstay of treatment of diabetic nephropathy is secondary prevention through tight blood pressure and glycaemic control, lipid management, and smoking cessation if appropriate (Box 13.6). Patients entering the symptomatic stage should be referred to and managed by a nephrologist, in addition to any follow-up occurring in primary care. Good communication between primary and secondary care is important to achieve the best outcomes and the best use of specialist expertise.

Angiotensin-converting enzyme inhibitors (ACEIs)

Angiotensin-converting enzyme inhibitors (Box 13.7) have been shown to reduce progression of diabetic nephropathy, and they should be offered to all patients with any degree of albuminuria, even if the blood pressure is normal. They reduce the risk of end stage renal failure requiring dialysis or transplantation, and improve all-cause mortality. Patients may fail to tolerate ACEIs for a number of reasons. A cough is a relatively common side-effect and requires substitution of the drug with an angiotensin 2 receptor blocker.

Box 13.6 Treatment Targets in Diabetic Nephropathy

Treatment targets in diabetic nephropathy should be individually tailored, but generally aim for:

- Blood pressure <130/80
- HbA1c <6.5% (48 mmol/mol)
- Total cholesterol <4.0 mmol/l and LDL <2.0 mmol/l
- Non-smoker status

In established nephropathy with proteinuria, it is safe to assume that the patient has widespread microvascular and macrovascular (including coronary artery) disease.

Box 13.7 Currently Available Angiotensin-Converting Enzyme Inhibitors (ACEIs) and Angiotensin 2 Receptor Blockers

ACEIs	Angiotensin 2 receptor blockers
Ramipril	Candesartan
Lisinopril	Valsartan
Enalapril	Losartan
Captopril	Irbesartan
Trandolapril	Telmisartan
Quinapril	Eprosartan
Perindopril	Olmesartan
Cilazapril	
Fosinopril	
Moexipril	

Box 13.8 Every Effort should be Made to Help the Patient to Tolerate ACEI or A2RB

ACE inhibition is a vital component of the secondary prevention of diabetic nephropathy. All too often, ACEIs are withdrawn due to minor side effects, without considering other management options, denying the patient the opportunity to benefit in the long term from this therapy. Sometimes the patient does not appreciate the potential benefits and, too readily, opts for other means of blood pressure control.

If a cough occurs with ACEI, offer an A2RB, which will not cause a cough.

If other side effects occur, review the schedule and adjust other medication accordingly:

- *Dizziness.* Is the patient also taking diuretics? Do they really need them at this dose? Are they fluid-depleted? Even though the symptom may have been precipitated by the addition of ACEI, it may be resolved by withdrawal of other drugs such as a thiazide or a beta blocker instead of the ACEI. Angiotensin-converting enzyme inhibitors sometimes produce a 'first dose hypotension' effect but, provided renal function has not deteriorated, it may be safe to continue by giving the drug before bed, unless the patient is at risk of night-time falls. Clearly, this advice needs to be tailored to the individual. Start at the lowest possible dose and titrate upwards, monitoring blood pressure and renal function.
- *Deterioration in renal function.* Consider withdrawal of diuretics prior to commencing ACE inhibition, and check blood pressure and renal function before and soon after starting therapy and after each dose increase. If a decline in e-GFR occurs, consider other drugs that may be contributing, such as non-steroidal anti-inflammatory drugs (NSAIDs), and review the need for them rather than withdrawing the ACEI unless this is really necessary.

Even a small dose of ACEI is better than nothing.

For those who really cannot tolerate ACEIs, tight blood pressure control with other agents is still a priority

These drugs have also been shown to reduce progression to end stage renal failure, but not all-cause mortality, and ACEIs are still the preferred option if tolerated (Box 13.8).

Lipid management and aspirin

Patients with established proteinuria due to diabetic nephropathy are at high risk of cardiovascular events, and justify the same approach to cardiovascular risk reduction as those with known coronary artery disease. In addition to lipid-lowering agents (which are recommended anyway for most people with diabetes), this includes aspirin in a high proportion of patients, particularly those with established CVD. Aspirin sometimes has an adverse effect on renal function but, at low dose, the benefits may outweigh this risk, provided GFR is greater than 15 ml/min. See Chapter 6 for more on the use of aspirin in selected patients.

Protein restriction

There is a role for protein restriction in diabetic nephropathy, but this is generally recommended only if intake is excessive. Orally ingested protein increases urea production and places a strain on the kidneys, exacerbating uraemia in the later, symptomatic stages. At earlier stages, there is some evidence that protein restriction reduces the decline in GFR, but this effect is minor and restriction is not recommended, unless the protein intake is particularly high. Assessment by a dietician working in collaboration with the nephrologist is useful to clarify this in each individual case.

Referral to secondary care

Early nephropathy is likely to be identified in primary care and, for much of the course of the disease, management based in primary care is appropriate in order to maintain tight control of blood pressure (with ACEIs or A2RB), blood glucose and lipids. Liaison with secondary care is important, as well as clearly understood thresholds for referral to a nephrologist.

Secondary care expertise is important at the stages where the patient has become symptomatic, and particularly as they progress towards dialysis dependence and develop further nephrological complications, including secondary hyperparathyroidism with osteomalacia. Access to secondary care varies depending on the health care infrastructure available. In the UK, it is usual to refer patients whose e-GFR has fallen below 25 ml/min, those with symptoms of uraemia, or those with other complications.

Other problems

Acute

Patients with established nephropathy may develop acute problems that require prompt action. Practitioners caring for such patients must be aware of the necessary action required. The detailed management of these is beyond the scope of this book, but we include here some important examples.

Hyperkalaemia. Potassium levels are prone to rise with declining renal function and are liable to rise further in response to ACEI or A2RBs. Such patients require close monitoring. Levels rising above 5.7 mmol/l require prompt action, and those above 6 mmol/l are an emergency, due to risk of fatal arrhythmias.

Acute deterioration in renal function. This may occur for a number of reasons, and is more likely in a patient with already compromised renal function. Causes may be pre-renal (e.g. dehydration or shock from any cause), renal (including drug therapy, sepsis, myoglobinaemia), or post-renal (e.g. obstruction due to retention or by tumour). The patient should be transferred urgently to secondary care, their hydration status assessed, precipitating factors identified, and the need for urgent dialysis or other support determined.

Overwhelming infection. Patients with diabetic nephropathy are at higher risk from ascending urinary infection, which may cause not only an acute pyelonephritis and septicaemia, but also an acute papillary necrosis with further decline in renal function. Urinary infection must be actively managed and, if there is evidence of involvement of the kidneys, this should be undertaken in hospital with intravenous antibiotics.

More gradual

More gradual decline in renal function. This may occur in patients taking over-the-counter NSAIDs without their clinician's awareness and, occasionally, patients taking statins may develop a low grade myositis, which is not reported but causes renal impairment due to undetected myoglobinaemia.

Secondary hyperparathyroidism. This is a complication of renal failure of any cause, and puts the patient at risk of osteomalacia and pathological fractures.

Erythropoietin deficiency

The normocytic anaemia associated with renal failure is caused partly by deficiency of the hormone erythropoietin (EPO), which is produced by the kidney and promotes erythrocyte production in the bone marrow. This anaemia tends to occur earlier in the course of nephropathy in diabetes than it does in other forms of renal disease. Treatment with replacement EPO injections is extremely effective, and can greatly improve quality of life. Other factors contributing to the anaemia, such as iron or folate deficiency, should be excluded prior to starting therapy (Box 13.9).

Box 13.9 **Treatment of Diabetic Nephropathy**

- Tight blood pressure control with ACEIs or A2RBs.
- Tight glycaemic control.
- Smoking cessation.
- Control of hyperlipidaemia if present.
- Protein restriction if intake excessive in the earlier stages, and for symptom relief later on.
- Erythropoietin for anaemia.
- Haemodialysis or continuous ambulatory peritoneal dialysis.
- Renal transplantation.

Prescribing issues in people with renal impairment

Numerous drugs must be used with caution in people with kidney disease, and some of these are particularly relevant to those with diabetes. They include drugs liable to worsen renal function, and those in which the renal impairment may make the drug unsafe. Some of these are described below, but this list is not comprehensive and only includes drugs particularly relevant to diabetes care. If in doubt, consult a formulary before prescribing any new drug to a patient with renal impairment.

Angiotensin-converting enzyme inhibitors (ACEIs). These drugs are an important (in fact, central) component of the treatment of diabetic nephropathy and, in the long run, should improve renal outcomes. However, in some cases, renal function may decline, particularly after the drug is first started, and this should always be done with close monitoring of renal function. A patient whose renal function deteriorates rapidly after the introduction of ACEI might have renal artery stenosis and may require investigation to exclude this. As mentioned above, it may be worth withdrawing other drugs, such as NSAIDs, in order to ensure that the patient tolerates the ACEI and, thereby, benefits from its long-term reno-protective effect.

Beta blockers. Certain beta blockers are excreted through the urine, and lower doses will be required. These include atenolol, nebivolol, celiprolol, acebutalol and sotalol.

Bezafibrate and gemfibrozil are similarly affected, and lower starting doses are appropriate. Bezafibrate should not be given if the creatinine clearance is less than 15 ml/min, and gemfibrozil if less than 30 ml/min.

Calcium channel blockers (CCBs). Some CCBs are affected by renal impairment, and doses may need to be adjusted accordingly or, in some cases, the drug avoided. Amlodipine and felodipine are unaffected.

Escitalopram, fluvoxamine and paroxetine. Depression is common in diabetes (see page 75), particularly where other chronic conditions such as renal failure are present, and antidepressants are likely to be offered to such patients. Many are safe, but the formulary should be consulted and some, such as escitalopram, fluvoxamine and paroxetine, carry cautions.

Insulin metabolism is affected by severe renal impairment, and this may require dose reductions as renal failure progresses.

Metformin is the only biguanide currently licensed for the treatment of diabetes. One of its adverse effects is lactic acidosis, and this is much more likely to occur in people with renal impairment. Past recommendations have been to avoid metformin in patients with a serum creatinine > 150 mcmol/l. Converting this advice to an e-GFR level is difficult as it depends on age and sex but, generally, a GFR level of 30 ml/min is appropriate, below which metformin should not be prescribed. A patient may have been taking metformin for a long time but, as renal function declines, this level may be reached and the drug should then be withdrawn and others used instead.

Nitrates should be used with caution in severe renal impairment.

Non-steroidal anti-inflammatory drugs (NSAIDs). Although not specific to diabetes care, these are commonly used drugs that may impair renal function and should be avoided if impairment is moderate or severe. If mild, these drugs may be used at the lowest effective dose, and with close monitoring of renal function. These side-effects are more likely if co-administered with ACEIs, and this interaction may mean that the patient is denied the benefits of ACEIs in order to preserve renal function.

Statins. Most patients with diabetes should be prescribed statins, and this particularly includes those with nephropathy, where control of lipid levels is a priority. Simvastatin, rosuvastatin and pravastatin are renally excreted, requiring lower doses, and atorvastatin may be a safer option in some patients, depending on the level of renal function.

Sulphonylureas. Some sulphonylureas are eliminated largely by the kidney, including glibenclamide and tolbutamide. Renal impairment will lead to prolonged duration of their effects, with risk of hypoglycaemia. Shorter-acting agents, including gliclazide, are now in more common use, and are largely metabolised without requiring renal clearance. Their use in patients with nephropathy is preferable, although doses may still need to be lowered.

Thiazide diuretics are relatively ineffective as diuretics if creatinine clearance is less that 30 ml/min. As antihypertensive drugs, they are not contraindicated in diabetes, but other options may be preferable in order to avoid aggravating hyperglycaemia and the hyperuricaemia associated with renal impairment.

Varenicline is a new drug prescribed to assist with smoking cessation, another important treatment of diabetic nephropathy. If creatinine clearance is less than 30 ml/min, then doses should be adjusted according to the manufacturers instructions.

Summary

The global rise in diabetes prevalence and improvements in cardio-vascular mortality are increasing the need for renal replacement therapy across the world, as rising numbers of patients (particularly type 2) survive to the end stage of renal failure. This trend will inevitably continue, requiring an expansion of the availability of dialysis and renal transplantation services. Programmes to prevent progression to the later stages of diabetic nephropathy are essential, and should be part of the organisational infrastructure of all primary care teams. Liaison between primary and secondary care and clear referral pathways are important to promote optimal outcomes and make the best use of specialist expertise.

Further reading and references

Rao A, *et al.* (2010) The Seventeenth Annual Report, Chapter 10. Bristol: UK Renal Registry.

Guidance. http://guidance.nice.org.uk/F.

SIGN Guidance. http://www.sign.ac.uk/pdf/sign103.pdf.

Van Dijk KJ, Jager B, Stengel C (2005). Renal replacement therapy for diabetic end-stage renal disease: Data from 10 registries in Europe (1991–2000). *Kidney International* **67**, 1489–1499.

CHAPTER 14

Eye Disease in Diabetes

Tim Holt[1] and Sudhesh Kumar[2]

[1]Nuffield Department of Primary Care Health Sciences, Oxford University, UK
[2]Warwick Medical School, University of Warwick; and WISDEM, University Hospital, Coventry, UK

OVERVIEW

- Diabetic retinopathy is still the leading cause of blindness in those under 65 years in industrialised countries.

- Early detection enables effective interventions to prevent visual loss.

- Screening for retinopathy should be available to all adult patients with diabetes.

- Screening programmes require effective coordination between primary care services, diabetologists and ophthalmologists.

- Patients with any degree of retinopathy require tight control of vascular risk factors.

- Other eye problems in diabetes include glaucoma, cataract, optic neuropathy and ocular palsies.

Introduction

Diabetic retinopathy is common, serious and costly, detectable in a pre-symptomatic phase, and treatable with widely available and effective interventions to prevent progression to disabling visual loss. Screening for retinopathy is, therefore, a priority area of diabetes care. Loss of vision is perhaps the complication that patients fear the most and, despite improving figures, this is still the commonest cause of blindness in working-age people in industrialised countries.

Modern ophthalmologic techniques, including laser therapy, commencing in the 1970s, have perhaps been the single most significant advance in the management of diabetes since the discovery of insulin. Widespread use of laser followed the US Diabetes Retinopathy Study (DRS), which first demonstrated its effectiveness in 1974.

Patients newly diagnosed with diabetes should be told about all the possible complications of their condition. In the case of retinopathy, there is a good chance that control of risk factors, combined with regular surveillance and early treatment of problems, will prevent future disability.

Screening techniques

As discussed in the chapter on surveillance (Chapter 12), all adult patients with diabetes should be offered retinopathy screening at diagnosis, and annually thereafter. This involves bilateral digital photography of both fundi following pupillary dilatation. A short-acting topical mydriatic, such as tropicamide 0.5% is usually used. A possible contra-indication is a history of acute angle-closure glaucoma, and caution should be applied in those with risk factors for this condition (older, hypermetropic patients), but serious problems are uncommon. Transient stinging of the eyes is to be expected, but is not serious. Visual acuity should be measured in both eyes prior to dilatation.

Early detection of changes (described below) should then be followed up through further assessment, more frequent review and treatment where indicated.

Pathogenesis

Diabetic retinopathy is largely a microvascular complication, involving disease in the small vessels, particularly of the basement membrane. Damage to these vessels results in increased permeability and leakage of blood or plasma into the extravascular space, with secondary thickening of the basement membrane. Disruption of the blood supply causes localised tissue hypoxia, triggering the release of vascular growth factors. It is these that promote the proliferation of new vessels during the later stages in both the retina and vitreous humour. Vascular insufficiency, due to atheroma of the larger vessels supplying the eye, or micro-emboli, from carotid artery disease, may further reduce tissue perfusion and oxygenation. Exudation and haemorrhage lead to fibrosis, further damaging visual function and predisposing to retinal detachment.

Background retinopathy

Risk of retinopathy correlates strongly with the duration of diabetes. Background changes are almost universal after 20 years of type 1 diabetes, and are frequently present at diagnosis in type 2 patients

ABC of Diabetes, Seventh Edition. Tim Holt and Sudhesh Kumar.

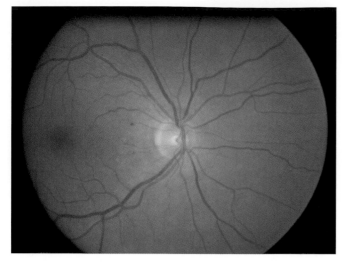

Figure 14.1 Background retinopathy with a few microaneurysms only. This stage is not likely to threaten vision in the near future, but tight control of vascular risk factors is important to reduce progression. Source: Photograph courtesy of Dr Sailesh Sankar.

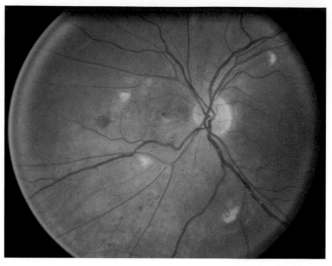

Figure 14.2 Pre-proliferative retinopathy with several 'cotton wool' spots, as well as background microaneurysms and blot haemorrhages. Source: Photograph courtesy of Dr Sailesh Sankar.

(Figure 14.1). The hallmark lesions are *microaneurysms*, which are visible on fundoscopy as minute 'dot' haemorrhages. Microaneurysms are not actually haemorrhages but are localised dilatations of capillaries. The small vessels themselves are typically too small to be detected, which results in the impression of an isolated haemorrhage. In contrast, 'blot' haemorrhages are, indeed, due to leakage of blood, usually into the nerve fibres above the basement membrane. They are noticeably larger and often irregular in outline.

Background changes do not cause visual loss, but do signify significant vascular disease and, particularly when occurring close to the visual axis, may require more frequent screening examinations.

Pre-proliferative retinopathy

Cotton wool spots

Localised ischaemia due to closure of diseased blood vessels results in a 'cotton wool' appearance (Figures 14.2 and 14.3), previously referred to as 'soft exudates', which is a misnomer as the process does not actually involve leakage or exudation. Such changes do not usually affect acuity themselves, but may herald the development of neovascularisation.

Hard exudates

Leakage of lipids from damaged capillaries leads to 'hard exudates' which, although not involving neovascularisation, may result in permanent visual loss through damage to the macula and fovea.

Venous beading and **intra-retinal microvascular abnormalities** (IRMAs) are further signs of pre-proliferative retinopathy.

Diabetic maculopathy

Increased permeability of the retinal vessels may result in localised oedema, even in the absence of exudates or new vessels (Figure 14.4). When this occurs at the macula, it can result in a very

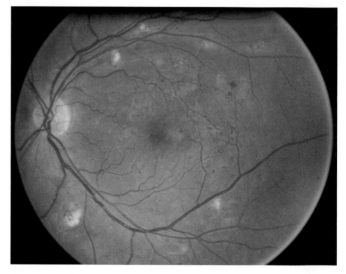

Figure 14.3 The same eye as in Figure 14.2, showing relative sparing of the macular region, but the retina is generally ischaemic and at risk of progression to sight threatening neovascularisation. Source: Photograph courtesy of Dr Sailesh Sankar.

acute deterioration in acuity over a period of hours. This complication is difficult to foresee but is treatable, so patients should be aware of the need to report changes in acuity, even if a recent screening examination was satisfactory. Exudative maculopathy may occur in a patient with more advanced pre-proliferative disease (Figure 14.5).

Proliferative retinopathy

The more serious forms of diabetic retinopathy, associated with permanent visual loss, are usually the result of failure of preventive interventions, allowing proliferative changes involving new vessel growth (Figure 14.6).

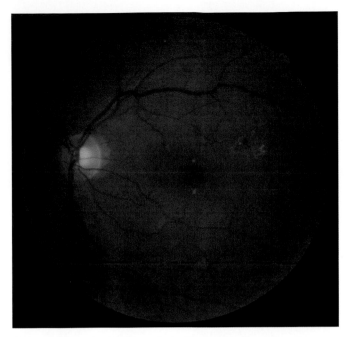

Figure 14.4 Maculopathy in a patient with established background changes, indicated by microaneurysms and blot haemorrhages. Source: Photograph courtesy of Dr Sailesh Sankar.

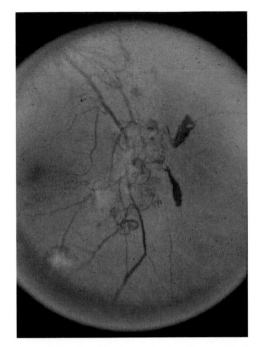

Figure 14.6 Proliferative diabetic retinopathy showing new vessel formation and vitreous haemorrhages. Source: Photograph courtesy of Dr Sailesh Sankar.

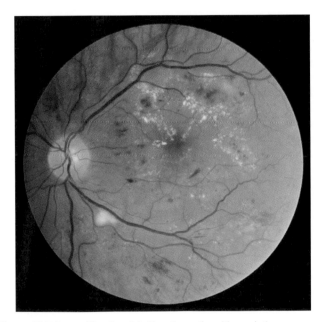

Figure 14.5 Pre-proliferative diabetic retinopathy with exudative maculopathy. At least two cotton wool spots indicate retinal ischaemia. There are multiple microaneurysms and haemorrhages, venous beading, and both linear and stellate exudates at the macula, with arterio-venous nipping due to coexisting hypertension. Source: Photograph courtesy of Dr Paul O'Hare and Dr Vinod Patel.

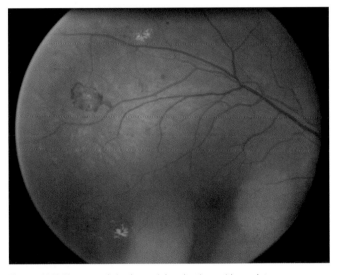

Figure 14.7 New vessels in the peripheral retina, with exudates. Source: Photograph courtesy of Dr Sailesh Sankar.

Neovascularisation

Figure 14.7 shows the typical appearance of new vessel formation. These develop in response to vascular growth factors released in response to tissue hypoxia in the basement membrane. In contrast to macular oedema, these changes usually develop gradually and progressively, providing opportunities for prevention. It is unusual for neovascularisation to develop without a recognisable pre-proliferative phase. If preventive measures fail, neovascularisation may result in permanent loss of acuity or visual field.

Sequelae of new vessel growth

New vessels usually arise on the venous side of the circulation and are not normal vessels –they are friable and bleed easily, resulting in vitreous haemorrhage and irreversible fibrosis of the surrounding

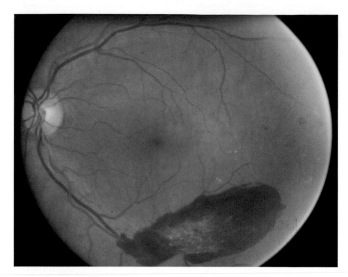

Figure 14.8 Extensive haemorrhage into the subhyaloid layer between the retina and the vitreous humour, resulting from proliferative retinopathy. Source: Photograph courtesy of Dr Sailesh Sankar.

tissues (Figure 14.8). This fibrosis causes traction on the underlying retina, promoting retinal detachment, with accumulation of fluid between the neural and pigmented layers.

Further assessment of established retinopathy

Microaneurysms are commonly detected on screening examinations, and usually require no immediate action other than attention to risk factors, particularly glycaemic control. Patients should be aware of the importance of attending future examinations but, unless the background changes are close to the macula, annual follow-up will probably be appropriate. Pre-proliferative changes, particularly when close to the visual axis, require further assessment with an ophthalmologist, preferably one with an interest in diabetic eye disease.

In addition to slit lamp examination and retinal photography, a number of techniques are used to further evaluate the eye in diabetes.

Fluorescein angiography may be used to highlight small vessels that are otherwise too small to see. This helps in the assessment of the microcirculation and can distinguish (for instance) between generalised venous dilatation and venous beading, the latter being much more significant prognostically and associated with closure of the surrounding capillary circulation. It helps to distinguish new vessels from normal vessels, which typically form a branching pattern like a tree, while abnormal new vessels frequently join up with themselves again to form arcs or networks of vessels called 'rete'. Fluoroscein angiography can also distinguish cotton wool spots (which are ischaemic areas of underperfusion) from areas associated with haemorrhage and exudation.

Ocular coherence tomography may be useful to determine the presence of traction on the macula in a patient with maculopathy (Figure 14.9), as this condition also involves oedema, and the relative contribution of each is not always evident on slit lamp examination or photography.

Measurement of intra-ocular pressure is important in the assessment of anyone with established retinopathy, particularly those with proliferative retinopathy. Peripheral new vessels may be missed on screening examinations, and are often associated with rubeosis iridis, predisposing to secondary glaucoma (see below).

Treatment options

Treatment of retinopathy depends largely on the stage of the disease, but also on other factors, including the location. A distinction is made between new vessels at the disc (NVD) and new vessels elsewhere (NVE).

Pre-proliferative changes usually only require tightening control of vascular risk factors, although maculopathy may require laser treatment, localised to the macula, to reduce leakage from blood vessels.

Pan-retinal photocoagulation

Proliferative retinopathy is caused by the release of vascular growth factors from ischaemic retinal tissue. Laser treatment destroys the upper layer to reduce the oxygen requirement of the ischaemic retina, thereby reducing the release of the factors that promote new vessel growth. For this to be effective, between 1000 and 2000 separate 'burns' may be required during a treatment course, and these are distributed all over the retina, particularly the peripheral areas (also known as 'scatter laser therapy'). This may reduce peripheral vision, but it is necessary to preserve the function of the visual axis (Figure 14.10). Not only is this treatment effective at reducing visual loss, it may also eventually improve acuity where this is reduced.

Vitrectomy

Haemorrhage into the vitreous humour may cause loss of acuity or of visual field, often of sudden onset. Alternatively, changes may be more gradual, due to secondary clouding and thickening of the usually transparent gel. Later scarring causes contracture with traction on the adjacent retina. Blood or other opaque tissue may be amenable to excision by vitrectomy, involving access to the vitreous via an incision in the sclera under local anaesthetic. The evacuated vitreous may be replaced with normal saline to maintain volume.

Other treatments

Intravitreous triamcinolone injection is sometimes offered to reduce leakage from diseased blood vessels, particularly when the macula is affected, but the procedure needs to be repeated recurrently as its benefits are not permanent. There is evidence that the lipid-lowering agent fenofibrate has a beneficial effect on retinopathy in type 2 diabetes, but the exact place for this drug in routine practice is still unclear.

Anti-vascular endothelial growth factor (VEGF)

There is increasing interest and use of intra-ocular anti-VEGF as a less destructive option to laser photocoagulation in vision threatening situations including macular oedema. They are used either as an adjunct, or in the place of laser therapy, but their place in current practice is still new. A useful review is provided by Gupta *et al.* (2013) and the evidence is also summarised in a NICE Technology Appraisal (2013).

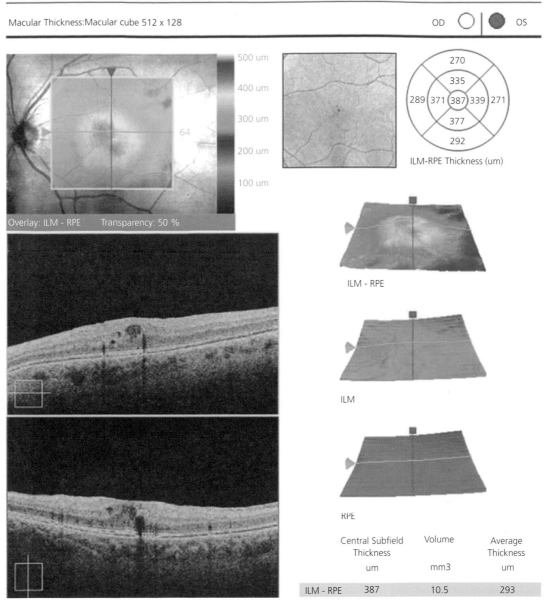

Figure 14.9 Ocular Coherence Tomography (OCT) has improved the assessment of diabetic retinopathy, and here demonstrates macular oedema. Source: Images courtesy of Mr Gary Misson.

Other eye problems in diabetes

Rubeotic glaucoma

Rubeosis is another name for the proliferation of blood vessels in response to growth factors triggered by hypoxia. When this occurs in the vessels of the anterior chamber, neovascularisation may disrupt the outflow of aqueous humour at the angle, causing a rise in intra-ocular pressure. This can lead, over time, to a secondary glaucoma, with damage to visual fields and acuity.

The screening programme for diabetic retinopathy in the UK does not include a measurement of intra-ocular pressure. However, people with diabetes are entitled to a free eye examination annually with a commercial optician, and pressure measurement should be offered during these assessments. Patients with evidence of

neovascularisation picked up during the screening programme will be referred on for further ophthalmological assessment, and pressure measurement will be provided in this setting. In addition to glaucoma that is secondary to rubeosis, people with diabetes are more prone to primary chronic (open angle) glaucoma than the general population.

Retinal detachment

This is a result of accumulation of fluid between the neural and pigmented retinal layers. As discussed above, fibrosis of the vitreous humour next to the retina promotes this process, particularly in those with established proliferative retinopathy. A peripheral detachment may produce a field defect of gradual or sudden onset. This may or may not be noticed by the patient, but it is typically

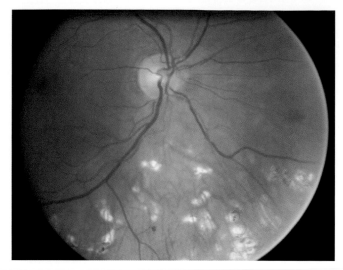

Figure 14.10 Scarring resulting from laser therapy in the peripheral retina. Source: Photograph courtesy of Dr Sailesh Sankar.

heralded by a sensation of bright flashing lights. Traction, with or without actual detachment, may affect the macula (as discussed above) to produce acute deterioration in acuity.

Cataract

Cataract is common in diabetes, and is worsened by poor glycaemic control. The treatment is the same as for the general population.

Retinal vein occlusion

The retinal vein may become occluded, particularly if hyperglycaemia is sufficient to produce hyperviscosity. Occlusion of the central retinal vein causes catastrophic unilateral loss of vision or, more commonly, a branch retinal occlusion causes loss of visual field. Associated haemorrhage, oedema and closure of the capillary circulation are typical and complicate the picture. Fluoroscein angiography may help to determine whether spontaneous resolution is likely, or whether focal laser treatment to seal off leaking vessels is required.

Diabetic optic neuropathy

This is a rare complication of diabetes, causing swelling and loss of function of the optic nerve, with progressive loss of acuity.

Ocular muscle palsies

People with diabetes may develop an ocular muscle palsy as an acute or subacute neuropathic event. This classically affects the third cranial (oculomotor) nerve, producing an outward and downward gaze, due to weakness of adduction and unopposed action of the superior oblique. There may be an associated ptosis. In diabetes where the cause is ischaemic, the pupillary reflex may be spared.

Living with diabetic retinopathy

Patients whose acuity or visual field is permanently affected require a lot of support. The first issue concerns driving ability and other safety issues. The Driving and Vehicle Licensing Authority (DVLA) issue regularly updated guidance on the medical standards of fitness to drive. For those more seriously affected, low vision clinics are available to help manage everyday self-care and promote independence. Loss of role in the home, the workplace and in society at large is potentially devastating, and requires a proactive approach to individual support in order to minimise the impact on quality of life.

Summary

Modern ophthalmological techniques, including laser therapy, represent a major victory in the ongoing battle against diabetes. Combined with effective retinopathy screening programmes, they are progressively reducing the risk of visual loss. Liaison between primary and secondary care, clearly defined referral pathways and patient education are vital if the benefits of these techniques are to be maximised.

The assessment of visual symptoms in diabetes is complex, and patients must have ready access to specialist expertise for the assessment of any unexpected change in acuity. The infrastructure required to provide high-quality care is, largely, only available in industrialised countries; meanwhile, diabetes prevalence is escalating elsewhere. Responding to this escalation and its impact on the visual health of the global community is a major challenge for the coming decades.

Further reading and references

DVLA. 'At a glance' Guide to medical standards of fitness to drive. Available at: http://www.dvla.gov.uk/medical/ataglance.aspx

Early Treatment of Diabetic Retinopathy Study Group (1985). Photocoagulation for diabetic macular edema. Early Treatment Diabetic Retinopathy Study. Archives of Ophthalmology 103, 1796–1806.

Gupta N, Mansoor S, Sharma A et al. (2013). Diabetic Retinopathy and VEGF. The Open Ophthalmology Journal 7, 4–10.

National Institute for Health and Care Excellence (2013). Ranibizumab for treating diabetic macular oedema (TA 237). London.

Noonan JE, Jenkins AJ, Ma JX, Keech AC, Wang JJ, Lamoureux EL (2013). An update on the molecular actions of fenofibrate and its clinical effects on diabetic retinopathy and other microvascular end points in patients with diabetes. Diabetes 62(12), 3968–3975.

The Diabetic Retinopathy Vitrectomy Study Research Group (1985). Early vitrectomy for severe vitreous hemorrhage in diabetic retinopathy. Two-year results of a randomized trial. Archives of Ophthalmology 103(11), 1644–1652.

The Wisconsin Epidemiologic Study of Diabetic Retinopathy (1994). XIV. Ten-year incidence and progression of diabetic retinopathy. Archives of Ophthalmology 112, 1217–1228.

CHAPTER 15

The Diabetic Foot

Tim Holt[1], Gurdev Deogon[2] and Sudhesh Kumar[2]

[1]Nuffield Department of Primary Care Health Sciences, Oxford University, UK
[2]Warwick Medical School, University of Warwick; and WISDEM, University Hospital, Coventry, UK

OVERVIEW

- Foot complications of diabetes are common and include arterial insufficiency and peripheral neuropathy, which can readily lead to ulceration.

- Foot ulcers may be associated with deep infection and put the patient at risk of osteomyelitis and systemic sepsis.

- Maintaining foot health demands a proactive approach, involving regular checks and patient education, which should be part of routine surveillance.

- Development of an 'at risk' foot justifies more frequent assessment.

- Conservative measures include removal of callus, desloughing, pressure relief casts, surgical debridement, abscess drainage and revascularisation.

- Local care pathways for managing foot complications should be well understood in order to ensure prompt action and reduce the need for amputation.

Introduction

Foot complications are a serious threat to patients with diabetes (Figure 15.1) and must always be treated energetically. Three major factors are vascular disease, peripheral neuropathy and a raised risk of infection. These may threaten not only the limb in question, but also the life of the individual, and regular surveillance and early intervention are essential. In particular, when acute problems arise, such as tissue breakdown and subsequent infection, prompt referral and appropriate management by an experienced multidisciplinary team are key to ensuring improved outcomes in this cohort.

Around 50% of non-traumatic foot amputations are carried out on people with diabetes. Advanced stage foot disease leads to considerable morbidity, psychosocial burden and, indeed, coupled with co-morbidity is associated with a high mortality. Foot problems are perhaps the most preventable complication of diabetes, but necessitate carefully thought-out integrated working and locally agreed

care pathways with experienced hospital interdisciplinary teams. They require, above all, healthcare professionals at each level with the necessary skill sets to identify patients at risk, knowledge of whom to refer and the importance of good communication. Equally, education and prevention strategies should be interwoven into the strategic fabric for local foot care provision. This includes embedding a programme of education for the patient and, indeed, their carers, bearing the sometimes debilitating consequences of this often insidious condition.

The three key risk factors

Vascular insufficiency

Peripheral vascular disease is often asymptomatic until a well-established stage. Classic early symptoms of intermittent claudication pain can easily be masked with concomitant neuropathy. Ischaemia reduces the immunological response to infection, delays healing and raises the likelihood of anaerobic infection in the deeper tissues.

It is important to highlight that the purely ischaemic foot in diabetes has been previously considered to be fairly rare (often noted at around 10% of cases). With medical advances and increasing longevity of patients living with diabetes, the prevalence of peripheral vascular disease will continue to increase in this cohort.

Neuropathy

Peripheral neuropathy reduces light touch sensation putting the foot at risk of unnoticed trauma. Pain is an innate protective mechanism and its loss makes the patient vulnerable to repetitive trauma and significant injury. Neuropathy also impairs proprioception and, coupled with denervation of intrinsic musculature of the foot, leads to deformity and swelling of the joints. In cases of advanced foot pathology, these problems can mask deeper foot sepsis, which should always be suspected when apparently superficial infection fails to heal.

Neuropathy is extremely common (up to 50% of type 2 patients) but, in many of these, it produces no symptoms and can only be

ABC of Diabetes, Seventh Edition. Tim Holt and Sudhesh Kumar.

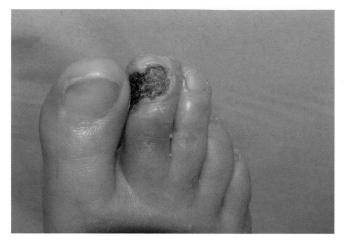

Figure 15.1 Necrotic ulcer on the second toe, with proximal erythema and swelling. Source: Photograph courtesy of Mr G S Deogon.

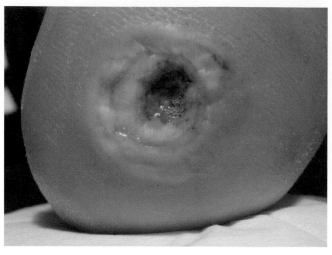

Figure 15.2 Deep heel ulceration in a neuropathic foot.

excluded through physical examination. Autonomic neuropathy is less common, but may cause reduction in sweating, with dryness of the skin, promoting fissuring and ulceration. Intrinsically autonomic neuropathy leads to arteriovenous shunting, which is clinically discernable through venous distension of the veins on the dorsum of the foot and lower calf.

Infection

Infection has often been described as the great destroyer[1]. It may be obvious superficially, or may be deeper, where it can invade bone, form abscesses, promote gangrene and produce systemic sepsis.

> 'While mild infections are relatively easily treated, moderate infections may be limb threatening, and severe infections may be life threatening.'
>   International Diabetes Federation Consensus Guidelines on the Management and Prevention of the Diabetic Foot, 2003.

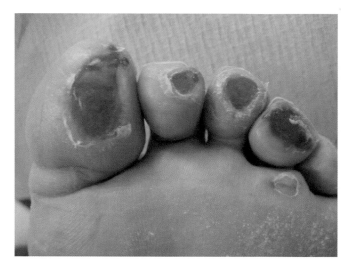

Figure 15.3 Pressure from tight footwear on insensitive toes has caused calluses now ulcerating superficially.

Patterns of presentation

Although the factors often co-exist, two major patterns are seen (all photographs courtesy of Mr G S Deogon, WISDEM Diabetes Foot Clinic, University Hospital, Coventry).

The neuropathic foot

Where neuropathy predominates, the problems tend to occur at the pressure areas on the plantar surfaces, and ulcers are usually preceded by callus formation on the sole. Neuropathic feet (Figures 15.2 and 15.3) are typically warm, with easily palpable pulses, due to reduction of sympathetic tone on the arteries, but reduced sensation is present on microfilament testing. Toe deformities, pronounced extensor tendons and an exacerbated medial longitudinal

arch may be present, along with swelling of the joints (Charcot's joints). Occasionally, severe neuropathy may cause oedema of the feet and lower legs. Deformity and swelling alone in the absence of properly accommodating and supporting footwear can often be the precipitating factor causing tissue injury in the neuropathic foot.

The ischaemic or neuro-ischaemic foot

Where arterial insufficiency is the major factor, the foot is often cool to the touch and pulses are reduced or absent. Ironically, the presence of a bounding pulse can also lend false confidence, due the presence of autonomic denervation, causing arterio-venous shunting. Therefore, clinical examination should always take into account a range of indicators, including the overall temperature and skin colour.

Hair growth may be reduced, although this sign is rather non-specific in older patients. If ischaemia becomes critical, the foot is typically pink and painful, and urgent action is then required. Cyanosis is classically associated with purple discolouration.

[1] Prof Mike Edmonds, Kings College Hospital, London.

Ischaemic ulcers are usually distal and on the margins of the feet, rather than the soles (Figure 15.4). They are not necessarily related to callosities, in contrast to purely neuropathic ulcers. However, as alluded to previously, neuropathy and ischaemia frequently co-exist (the 'neuro-ischaemic foot', Figure 15.4), complicating assessment, and this overlap should always be borne in mind.

Regular surveillance

All patients with diabetes should have a thorough foot examination at least annually and, in those with signs of complications or 'at-risk' features, this frequency should be increased. The examination should include, as a minimum, the following:

- **Inspection of the general health of the feet**. Signs of deformity, hair loss, loss of skin integrity, loss of sweating, swelling of joints, callosities, nail health, fungal infection between the toes and in

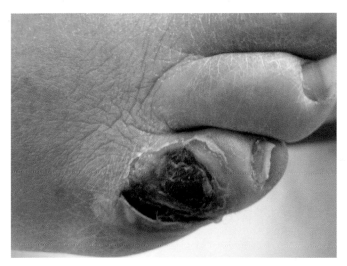

Figure 15.4 Gangrenous ulceration in a neuro-ischaemic foot.

the nails. Deformity or swelling may suggest an underlying Charcot's joint (see Figure 15.6). Callosities suggest abnormal distribution of weight over the sole, which may indicate peripheral neuropathy.
- **Assessment of vascular sufficiency**. Skin surface temperature and any unusual colour changes of the skin, detection of dorsalis pedis and posterior tibial pulses, capillary return at the toes.
- **Assessment of neurological integrity**. Light touch sensation using a 10 g nylon monofilament device at all of the 'at risk' areas (see Figure 15.5) and vibration sense at the great toe and ankle. Achilles tendon reflex.

Problems identified during a surveillance examination should be actioned accordingly (Boxes 15.1 and 15.2). Ulceration, however small, requires immediate active management. It is estimated that 4–10% of the population with diabetes has a foot ulcer. 85% of foot amputations in people with diabetes occur following the development of an ulcer.

If there are no acute problems requiring immediate action, then each foot should be classified according to its risk level, using the IDF risk categorisation system (Table 15.1 and Box 15.3). This can be used to determine the appropriate frequency of further examinations. Patient education should be offered at every routine check (Boxes 15.4, 15.5 and 15.6).

Charcot's joint

Loss of proprioceptive function leads to abnormal weight distribution in the ankle joint or the small joints of the foot. Initially, this produces wearing and degeneration at the articular surfaces, but later the joint may become distorted and dysfunctional. The initial presentation can simply be a hot and swollen foot. It can often be very difficult to differentiate these common symptoms from infection and, indeed, infection can coexist. With the difficulty of making an accurate diagnosis, an early referral to a specialist multidisciplinary team is strongly advised.

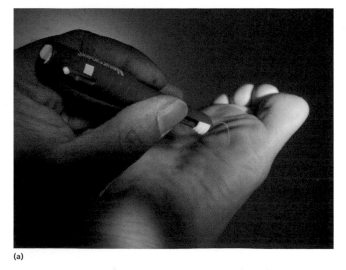

(a)

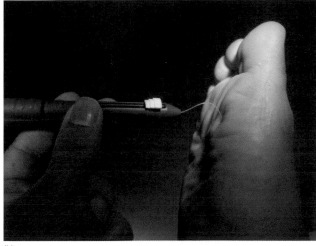

(b)

Figure 15.5 Patient having foot examined with 10 g monofilament. Source: Photographs courtesy of Mr G S Deogon.

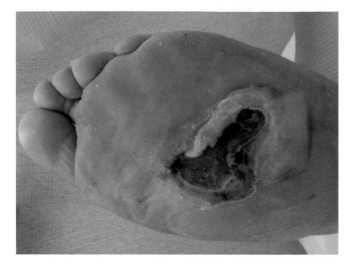

Figure 15.6 Classic Charcot's mid-foot ulcer, following collapse of the foot arches.

Box 15.1 Doppler Assessment

A suspicion of arterial insufficiency may be followed up by Doppler assessment to measure the Ankle Brachial Pressure Index (ABPI). This is a measure of the ratio of systolic pressures at the posterior tibial and brachial pulses. It should be carried out by professionals trained in the technique, and both inter- and intra-observer variability is a problem. Values greater than 1.0 are either normal or may suggest calcified vessels in the leg, particularly if greater than 1.2 (due to medial sclerosis raising the systolic pressure at the ankle). Values < 0.9 suggest ischaemia, and < 6.0 severe ischaemia. A Toe Brachial Pressure Index (TBPI) may be useful in cases of distal vessel disease.

Box 15.2 How Urgent is the Foot Problem?

Referral pathways should be organised with appropriate priority:

Callus on soles
Anaesthetic areas with
  no ulceration
Fungal infection
	Routine referral to specialist
	  podiatrist

Callus with evidence of haemorrhage	Urgent referral to podiatrist
Ulceration without infection	Referral to foot clinic within 48 hours

Ulceration with infection	Same day appointment at foot
	  clinic, or admission if there are
	  signs of systemic sepsis

Ischaemia

An absent foot pulse picked up at routine surveillance, with no symptoms or associated foot problems, should if considered significant and be followed up with reassessment every three months. Symptoms of vascular insufficiency (intermittent claudication, non-acutely cold foot) should trigger a 'soon' referral to a vascular surgeon. Rest pain requires an urgent same-day referral, and an acutely cold, painful, pulseless foot requires immediate transfer to hospital by ambulance 'nil by mouth'.

Table 15.1 IDF risk categorisation system for organising review intervals.

IDF Risk categorisation system		
Category	**Risk profile**	**Check-up frequency**
0	No sensory neuropathy	Once a year
1	Sensory neuropathy	Once every six months

2	Sensory neuropathy and
	  signs of peripheral
	  vascular disease and/or
	  foot deformities
		Once every three months

3	Previous ulcer	Once every 1–3 months

Box 15.3 IDF Risk Factors

- Previous ulcer/amputation.
- Lack of social contact.
- Lack of education.
- Impaired protective sensation (monofilaments).
- Impaired vibration perception.
- Absent Achilles tendon reflex.
- Callus.
- Foot deformities.
- Inappropriate footwear.

Box 15.4 International Diabetes Federation: Five Cornerstones of the Management of the Diabetic Foot

- Regular inspection and examination of the foot at risk
- Identification of the foot at risk
- Education of patient, family and healthcare providers
- Appropriate footwear
- Treatment of non-ulcerative pathology

From Apelqvist *et al.* (2008).

Box 15.5 Common Triggers for Ulceration

- Poorly fitting footwear.
- Unnoticed trauma from foreign body.
- Burns (hot bath, hot water bottle, radiator).
- Heel friction in a patient confined to bed.
- Nail infection.
- Dry skin.
- Self-treatment of callus with sharp instruments, or corn plasters.
- Callus not effectively treated.

The final stage of this process is a 'Charcot's joint', which is swollen and disfigured externally and disorganised internally. Reduced awareness of trauma, together with disordered movements, put the patient at high risk of secondary pressure ulceration, particularly if bespoke footwear with a correctly contoured planter interface is not provided. The internal arch of the foot falls, and ulceration at this site is common (Figure 15.6).

Treatment of diabetic foot complications

Importance of early referral

Once a problem is identified, the patient must access the necessary expertise for energetic treatment and follow-up through a well-designed and *locally effective* integrated foot care pathway, as recommended by national guidance (http://www.diabetes.org.uk/Documents/Professionals/Education%20and%20skills/Footcare-pathway.0212.pdf). This will usually involve a specialist multidisciplinary foot clinic and a community foot protection team, and all primary care clinicians must be clear regarding points of access, criteria and referral details.

The multidisciplinary foot clinic should have close links with surgical facilities, with rapid access to advanced orthotic, microbiological, radiological, vascular and orthopaedic specialties. A major cause of ulcers failing to heal is delay in starting appropriate treatment, by which time infection that might have been treated conservatively has penetrated the deeper tissues, causing necrosis and threatening the viability of the limb. Treatment options listed include both conservative and surgical approaches (Box 15.7).

Is the ulcer infected and if so, how severely?

The first decision is over whether or not a foot ulcer or wound is infected (Figure 15.7). Next, the depth and severity of infection must be assessed (Box 15.8). These answers will determine the need for antibiotics, the choice of antibiotic, the route of administration and setting in which they are given and the need and timing of surgical intervention, if appropriate. In addition to clinical examination, x-rays to exclude underlying osteomyelitis, and blood tests looking for leukocytosis or other inflammatory markers, may be required. However, patients with diabetes may not

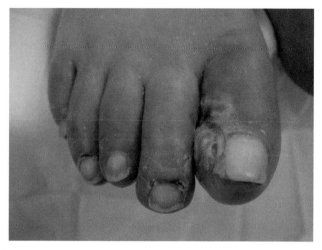

Figure 15.7 Neglected paronychia of the right great toenail with invasive infection and ulceration of proximal tissue.

produce the usual response to infection, and the absence of raised inflammatory markers does not exclude infection. Wound swab results should be interpreted carefully with clinical examination to distinguish between mere contamination or colonization and frank clinical infection.

Deep infection in the foot spaces must always be suspected whenever the patient does not respond to apparently appropriate therapy, when there are signs of systemic illness, or when signs of inflammation are present at some distance from the wound or ulcer.

Box 15.8 **Signs of Foot Wound Infection in Diabetes**

Local	Systemic	Radiographic
Pain	Fever	Osteomyelitis on x-ray
Tenderness	Rigors	
Eythema	Confusion	
Cellulitis	Hyperglycaemia	
Odour	Leukocytosis	
Necrosis	Raised inflammatory markers, e.g. C-reactive protein	
Gangrene		

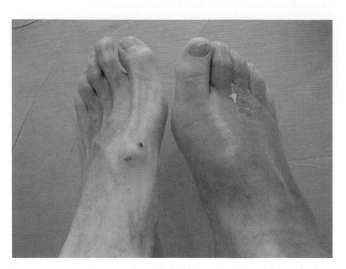

Figure 15.8 Extensive spreading cellulitis from a distal area of superficial ulceration.

Antibiotic therapy

Gram-positive organisms, including staphylococci and streptococci, are usually responsible for superficial foot infections, while deeper infection may be associated with more than one pathogen, including anaerobic and Gram-negative organisms (Figure 15.8). Treatment of a deep foot infection will usually require surgical removal of infected tissue, and antibiotics alone are unlikely to be adequate.

Identification of the responsible pathogen is important but will take time, and this should not delay the commencement of antibiotic treatment. Ideally, the infected tissue itself should be cultured following debridement but, by this time, the patient will usually have started empirical therapy, and swabs including actual pus if present (rather than ulcer slough) should be sent for microbiological analysis at the first opportunity. Antibiotic therapy is adjusted according to culture results, and may need to be continued until the ulcer has healed (Table 15.2 and Box 15.9).

Conservative management

Removal of callus

The finding of callus should lead to a referral to a podiatrist experienced in treating the feet of people with diabetes. In the absence of ulceration, this can be done less urgently, but the availability of this service is an essential component of the team management of diabetes.

> Under the UK's National Health Service, podiatry for diabetic feet (and other medical conditions) has become prioritised at the expense of general foot care in the older population without diabetes. This reflects the importance of professional treatment of early foot complications, including callus formation, which should never be 'self-managed'.

Desloughing of ulcers using maggots

Removal of the slough and debris at the base of a diabetic foot ulcer may be achieved using maggots (Figure 15.9). This may be more effective than other means of desloughing, and leaves the ulcer in a clean state ready to start healing.

Table 15.2 International Diabetes Federation: Suggested systemic antibiotic regimens for treating diabetic foot infections.

Severity of infection	Usual pathogen(s)	Potential regimens
Non-severe (oral for entire course)		
No complicating features	GPC	S-S pen; 1 G Ceph
Recent antibiotic therapy	GPC ± GNR	FQ, β-L-ase
Drug allergies		Clindamycin; FQ; T/S
Severe (intravenous until stable, then switch to oral equivalent)		
No complicating features	GPC2 ± GNR	β-L-ase; 2/3 G Ceph
Recent antibiotic/necrosis	GPC + GNR/ anaerobes	3/4 G Ceph; FQ + Clindamycin
Life-threatening (prolonged intravenous)		
MRSA unlikely	GPC + GNR + anaerobes	Carbapenem; Clindamycin Aminoglycoside
MRSA likely		Glycopeptide or linezolid + 3/4 G Ceph or FQ + metronidazole

Given at usual recommended doses for serious infections; modify for azotaemia, etc., based on theoretical considerations and available clinical trials. A high local prevalence of methicillin resistance among staphylococci may require using vancomycin or other appropriate anti-staphylococcal agents active against these organisms.
1 G Ceph – first generation cephalosporins (e.g. cephalexin, cefazolin);
2/3/4 G Ceph – 2nd/3rd/4th generation cephalosporins (e.g. cefoxitin, ceftazidime, cefepime);
β-L-ase – lactam-β lactamase-β inhibitor (e.g. amoxicillin/clavulanate, piperacillin/tazobactam);
FQ – fluoroquinolones (e.g. ciprofloxacin, levofloxacin);
GNR – gram-negative rod;
GPC – gram-positive cocci;
S-S pen – semi-synthetic (anti-staphylococcal) penicillin (e.g. flucloxacillin, oxacillin);
T/S – trimethoprim/sulfamethoxazole.
Carbapenem, e.g. imipenem/cilastatin, meropenem, ertapenem; aminoglycoside, e.g. gentamicin, tobramycin, amikacin; glycopeptides, e.g. vancomycin, teicoplanin.
Source: Reproduced with permission from the IDF International Consensus of the Diabetic Foot, the Practical Guidelines (1999) and Supplements (2003).

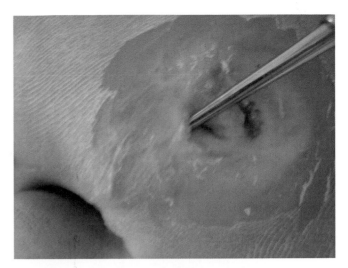

Figure 15.10 Probing a deep sinus beneath a neuropathic ulcer.

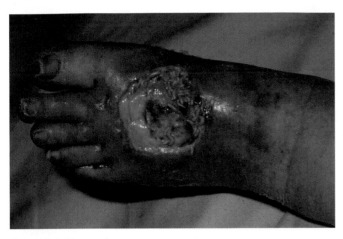

Figure 15.9 Maggot therapy.

Pressure relief casts

Ulcers often occur at the site of pressure, on the balls of the feet, the heel, or elsewhere on the sole. They are unlikely to heel if they continue to be exposed to this pressure. Scotchcast dressings with a hole over the ulcer are fitted to ensure that pressure is relieved in this area. It is essential that such casts are properly fitted, to avoid new ulcers forming elsewhere on the foot. Bed rest may also be necessary to assist healing, but immobility carries its own risk.

Surgical intervention

Debridement and abscess drainage

Surgical debridement is often required to remove necrotic tissue. This, in a sense, is a 'conservative' measure, in that it helps to reduce/prevent the need for amputation. Necrotic tissue acts like a foreign body, delaying healing, harbouring infection and making extension of infection, osteomyelitis and systemic sepsis more likely. In addition to debridement, other surgical measures include drainage of foot abscesses (which may require access to the deep foot spaces) (Figure 15.10).

Osteomyelitis, underlying infected, ulcerated skin is a common complication, and should be actively excluded through plain radiography (Figure 15.11) in all cases of deep or resistant infection. It often requires surgical excision and its presence will influence the choice, route of administration and duration of antibiotic therapy.

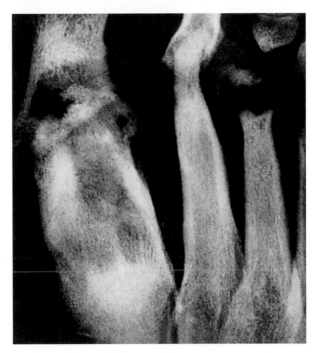

Figure 15.11 Radiograph of osteomyelitis.

Revascularisation and limb salvage

Revascularisation should, preferably, occur prior to the development of an ulcer in a patient with peripheral vascular disease (Figure 15.12). Often, however, ulceration is the first symptom of a silent background process. Where ulceration is established, angioplasty, bypass or reconstruction to the major vessels may greatly improve the chances of healing. Revascularisation is required urgently in the case of the critically ischaemic foot, requiring inpatient management.

Amputation

Amputation is indicated when conservative management fails, when persistent deep infection threatens systemic sepsis or progressive gangrene (Figure 15.13), or when rest pain is poorly

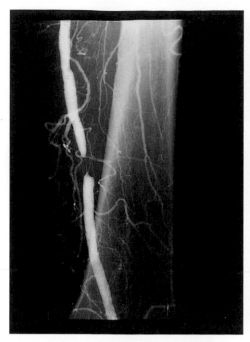

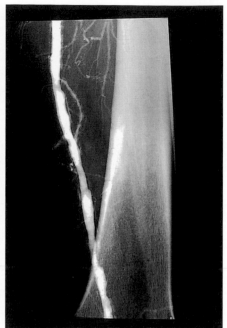

Figure 15.12 Radiograph of atheromatous narrowing.

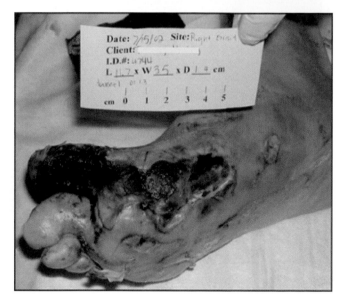

Figure 15.13 Extensive ulceration with infection and gangrene preceded this patient's below-knee amputation.

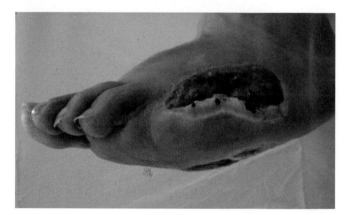

Figure 15.14 Clean wound following amputation of the left little toe. Note the callosities and neuropathic ulceration on the sole.

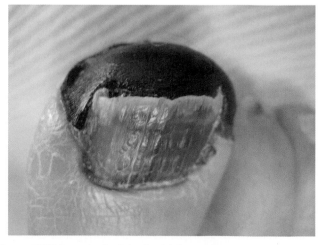

Figure 15.15 Dry necrosis of the distal right great toe.

controlled. When this is necessary, the limb must be assessed to determine the viability of proximal tissue. Adequate vascular supply is essential for healing and, if amputation is not extensive enough, this healing may fail. Toe amputation is usually unsuccessful when there is significant ischaemia present, but it may be an option in the purely neuropathic foot, or when revascularisation is successful (Figure 15.14). If so, conservation of the great toe may reduce the impact on limb function post-operatively. A dry, necrotic toe (Figure 15.15) may be left to 'auto-amputate' if infection is not an issue. Ensure that this is under close supervision of the multidisciplinary foot clinic.

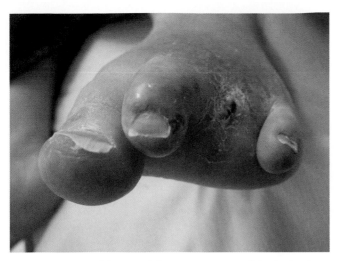

Figure 15.16 Successful healing following amputation of the third and fourth toes.

Rehabilitation

The patient must also be assessed in a more holistic way, to determine the options for rehabilitation. Some younger, fitter patients may manage with a prosthetic limb and regain walking mobility following limb amputation (Figure 15.16). Older, frailer or obese patients may not have this option, and are more likely to become wheelchair-dependent. These social consequences should be discussed with the patient and family if there is time before the decisions are made, even if amputation is inevitable.

The psychological response to amputation is complex. For some, it has been compared to a bereavement. Involvement of the patient and carers in management decisions helps in this adjustment. Apart from the human costs of amputation and resulting disability, the health economic effects justify an intensive, proactive approach to ulcer management and follow-up, even in countries with less developed resources.

Prognosis

Amputation often signifies the end stage of advanced complications, and amputees not only have a high risk of future amputation in the other limb, but also a high all-cause mortality rate in the year following the operation.

Further reading and references

Apelqvist J, Bakker K, van Houtum WH *et al.* (2008). Practical guidelines on the management and prevention of the diabetic foot: based upon the International Consensus on the Diabetic Foot (2007). Prepared by the International Working Group on the Diabetic Foot. *Diabetes/Metabolism Research and Reviews* 24(Suppl. 1), S181–S187.

International Diabetes Federation (2003). International consensus on the diabetic foot.

Jeffcoate W, Lipsky BA, Berendt AR *et al.*, on behalf of the three systematic review working parties of the International Working Group on the Diabetic Foot (2008). Unresolved issues in the management of ulcers of the foot in diabetes. *Diabetic Medicine* **25**, 1380–1389.

CHAPTER 16

Diabetic Neuropathy

Tim Holt[1] and Sudhesh Kumar[2]

[1]Nuffield Department of Primary Care Health Sciences, Oxford University, UK
[2]Warwick Medical School, University of Warwick; and WISDEM, University Hospital, Coventry, UK

OVERVIEW

- Diabetic neuropathy is a very common complication of diabetes.

- Peripheral neuropathy is often painful, and this is a disabling complication, increasing the risk of foot ulceration due to impaired sensation.

- Good control of hyperglycaemia, blood pressure and dyslipidaemia is important for prevention and reducing progression of neuropathy.

- Autonomic neuropathy causes a number of problems, including gastroparesis, gustatory sweating, postural hypotension and diarrhoea.

- Neuropathy may combine with vascular insufficiency to produce erectile dysfunction.

- Erectile dysfunction usually responds to drug therapy and other treatments.

Introduction

There are many forms of diabetic neuropathy, but the commonest form is a peripheral sensorimotor neuropathy that affects the feet first. Poorly controlled hyperglycaemia, uncontrolled hypertension and dyslipidaemia are associated with the development and progression of neuropathy. Excess alcohol consumption can also be a contributory factor. Chronic peripheral neuropathy due to diabetes is a progressive condition and can be expected to worsen over time. This is in contrast to acute neuropathies and especially cranial mononeuropathies, which tend to recover. Mononeuropathies result from microvascular disease. Compression neuropathies are also common in diabetes, and the commonest form of such neuropathy is carpal tunnel syndrome, although foot drop and ulnar neuropathy are also occasionally seen in patients with diabetes.

Peripheral neuropathy

Presentation

The commonest symptom is pain or altered sensation in the feet. Allodynia is common, and symptoms include a sensation of feet feeling cold or a feeling of pins and needles in the feet. Patients may complain that their bedclothes irritate the feet, and these symptoms may keep the patient up at night. In contrast, some patients experience a feeling of complete numbness. In both of these cases, reduced sensation in the feet is a hazard to the patient, who is then at risk of injury, ulceration and ensuing infection.

Neuropathy can affect both type 1 and type 2 patients. In patients with type 1 diabetes, it is seen after many years of diabetes. In type 2 patients, it may be present at the time of diagnosis itself. Patients on high doses of metformin may occasionally present with a neuropathy due to vitamin B12 deficiency; therefore, if in doubt, check serum vitamin B12.

During the early stages, clinical examination may not reveal any significant abnormality. Once clinically significant neuropathy is present, it is revealed by impairment of pressure perception tested with a 10 g monofilament, reduced vibration perception tested using a 128 Hz tuning fork, and absent ankle reflexes. Nerve conduction studies may reveal abnormalities in a significant proportion of patients with diabetes, who often do not have any symptoms and are not at high risk of foot ulceration. This test is more useful when compression neuropathy is suspected.

Tight control of glycaemia with insulin may reduce the progression of neuropathy. Several drugs have been developed and tested in trials, but none have so far been shown to alter the progression of neuropathy, other than control of diabetes and related risk factors.

Patients with peripheral neuropathy may also experience reduced sweating in the feet, which is a feature of autonomic dysfunction. The dryness of skin that results may predispose to foot ulceration. Regular application of intensive care Vaseline, or other skin emollients, help to keep the skin healthy.

ABC of Diabetes, Seventh Edition. Tim Holt and Sudhesh Kumar.

Treatment

Tight control of the principal risk factors, hyperglycaemia, blood pressure and lipids may help reduce progression. There is no specific therapy that has thus far proven to be effective in altering the natural history of neuropathy. Painful neuropathy can be extremely difficult to live with, and the clinician should be sympathetic to the plight of the patient and offer symptomatic treatment (Box 16.1). When it fails to respond to simple analgesics like paracetamol, tricyclic antidepressants, the antidepressant duloxetine, or anti-epileptic agents such as gabapentin or carbamazepine, may be helpful. Opiates may sometimes be required for pain that does not respond to other measures.

Acute painful neuropathies

These tend to present acutely and recover over the course of 6-18 months. They are more commonly seen in patients with type 2 diabetes, and are thought to be due to vascular disease. Effective pain relief is required, as is good control of glycaemia and associated risk factors. Application of Opsite may help to relieve pain in these cases.

Autonomic neuropathy

Autonomic neuropathy occurs as a long-term complication of diabetes and is associated with long duration of diabetes and a history of poor glycaemic control.

Postural hypotension

Even in those with a clinically detectable drop in blood pressure of more than 20 mm Hg, symptoms are unusual. A drop in blood pressure of more than 30 mm Hg is often seen in those patients who complain of dizziness while standing. The patient's blood pressure should be checked at least two minutes after standing from a supine position. Unexplained hypoglycaemia and new onset of postural hypotension may also be due to Addison's disease in patients with type 1 diabetes. When suspected, this diagnosis should be excluded by a short synacthen test.

For patients with symptoms, the treatment should start with exclusion of drugs that can aggravate the problem. Where there are significant symptoms, it may be necessary to ask the patient to increase salt intake. Fludrocortisone may be prescribed for symptomatic postural hypotension after the above measures have been tried.

Gustatory sweating

Profuse facial sweating, especially after eating something savoury, is a symptom of autonomic neuropathy. Often, an explanation is all that is needed but, if treatment is required, glypyrrolate cream can be prepared for the patient by any hospital pharmacy department. The cream is then applied to the affected areas.

Autonomic diarrhoea

Nocturnal diarrhoea in patients with long-standing diabetes may be due to autonomic neuropathy. Here, exclusion of other bowel problems, especially conditions such as coeliac or pancreatic disease, is important. Autonomic neuropathy can be established by testing for cardiovascular autonomic dysfunction (Figure 16.1). Treatment can be given in the form of codeine phosphate, but doxycycline 50 mg given daily for 3–4 days, and thereafter once every other day for two weeks is often effective in many patients.

Diabetic gastroparesis

Gastroparesis, leading to vomiting, is rare, although milder forms are not uncommon. Patients may report vomiting the contents of meals consumed more than 24 hours earlier. Presence of a gastric splash on examination is another clue to the diagnosis. The patient should then be referred for investigation, and radiolabelled porridge studies can help establish the diagnosis.

Pro-kinetic anti-emetics are often used, including metoclopramide. In severe cases, where the patient suffers intractable vomiting, percutaneous endoscopic jejunostomy may be required.

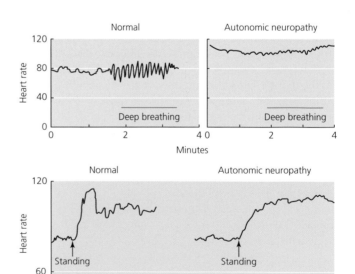

Figure 16.1 Heart rate changes in a normal subject (left) and a patient with autonomic neuropathy (right), showing loss of heart rate variation in autonomic neuropathy during deep breathing, at six breaths a minute (top), and loss of 'overshoot' cardiac acceleration on standing (bottom).

Box 16.1 **Treatment Options for Painful Neuropathy**

Topical agents:
- Topical capsaicin cream.
- Opsite dressing to reduce contact pain.
- Lignocaine-impregnated patches (Versatis).

Oral agents:
- Simple analgesia (e.g. paracetamol).
- Amitriptyline (10-25 mg at night, increased if needed up to 75 mg).
- Duloxetine 60-120 mg daily.
- Pregabalin (150 mg/day in two to three divided doses, increased if needed after 3-7 days to 300 mg/day in two to three divided doses, then further increased if needed after seven days to maximum 600 mg/day in two to three divided doses).
- Gabapentin (300 mg on day one, then 300 mg twice a day on day two, then 300 mg three times a day on day three, increased according to response in steps of 300 mg/day to maximum 1.8 g daily).
- Carbamazepine, sodium valproate, topiramate.
- Opiates if pain intractable (but high risk of dependency).

Other autonomic neuropathic problems

Severe constipation, requiring colectomy, is now exceptionally rare, but is still seen from time to time. Other complications due to autonomic neuropathy may include neurogenic bladder, resulting in urinary retention. This may eventually require treatment by self-catheterisation, two to three times daily. Erectile dysfunction and retrograde ejaculation are also problems related to autonomic neuropathy. Respiratory arrests may also occur. This is important when patients undergo surgery with anaesthesia.

Erectile dysfunction

Erectile dysfunction is common in men over the age of 50 years. In men with diabetes, it is more common and occurs at a younger age, causing considerable distress both to the patient and to his partner. Neuropathy, vascular disease, alcohol and drugs are the main underlying organic causes for erectile dysfunction in patients with diabetes. However, as in those without diabetes, in many it has an underlying psychogenic basis. The anxiety that this loss of function is due to diabetes makes the problem worse.

Clinical assessment

Patients complaining of erectile dysfunction should undergo a full clinical examination, including examination of the external genitalia. Gradual onset of erectile dysfunction, with loss of nocturnal erections, in someone with long-standing diabetes is likely to be due to diabetes. On the other hand, sudden onset and intermittent symptoms and the preservation of nocturnal erections suggest an underlying psychological basis instead. In these cases, exploring any difficulties in the patients' relationships, or any major work or financial stress, may reveal the underlying reason. The presence of neuropathy, peripheral and/or autonomic makes neurogenic impotence more likely. The presence of significant vascular disease suggests that there may be vascular insufficiency. Many drugs taken with diabetes can cause erectile dysfunction, and excess alcohol intake is often a significant contributor to the problem. Symptoms and signs of hypogonadism should also be looked for.

Investigation

Thyroid function tests and free testosterone should be checked. Serum prolactin should be measured if free testosterone is low. These tests are usually normal in patients with diabetes and erectile dysfunction. In patients with normal serum testosterone, there is no value in prescribing testosterone supplements, although patients may often request this.

Management of erectile dysfunction

First, it is important to explain the cause to the patient and his partner, and also to provide reassurance that it can usually be effectively treated. This is especially important if no obvious underlying cause is found and psychological factors are thought to be likely to have caused the symptom. Patients with major psychological problems that have been identified during the consultation, or with significant relationship problems may benefit from being referred to a psychologist or relationship counsellor.

Phosphodiesterase inhibitors

First line drug treatment includes oral therapies such as phosphodiesterase inhibitors. Many men can be successfully treated with oral therapy such as Sildenafil, Vardenafil or Tadalafil. The patient is asked to take the tablet between 30 minutes to one hour before sexual activity if using Sildenafil, while some preparations can be taken up to 24 hours earlier (Tadalafil). These treatments are contra-indicated in those taking nitrates, those with blood pressure < 90/50 mmHg, or after a recent stroke or myocardial infarction. The success of Sildenafil and other oral agents has revolutionised the treatment of erectile dysfunction and has improved the lives of millions with diabetes.

Sublingual apomorphine

This is rapidly absorbed after sublingual administration and acts as a dopamine agonist. It is effective within 10–20 minutes but requires sexual stimulation to be effective. The dose ranges between 2–3 mg and it is effective in approximately 50% of diabetic patients suffering from erectile dysfunction.

Prostaglandin preparations

Transurethral alprostadil (MUSE). This is applied into the urethra with an applicator provided. Recently, a urethral cream (Vitaros) has become available that works within 5–30 minutes. This modality of treatment can produce an erection after sexual stimulation.

Intracavernosal injection: alprostadil. This is less widely used since the oral therapies have become available. However, it is used as second line therapy after oral therapies have proved ineffective. Many diabetes centres and hospital neurology departments offer a service where patients are taught how to give themselves an injection avoiding the penile artery and the urethra. Bruising and priapism may complicate this therapy.

Vacuum devices

These devices have become less widely used with the availability of other therapies. However, it is an option where pharmacological therapies have failed, or when venous leak is a problem. Several companies now produce vacuum devices, and the patient is usually required to purchase the device. The external cylinder is fitted over the penis, a vacuum is created inside the cylinder, resulting in penile engorgement and, at this point, an elastic ring is applied to the base of the penis that sustains the erection. This form of therapy is more often used in older patients.

Penile prostheses

Various prostheses are available that are surgically inserted into the shaft of the penis. Some sophisticated devices allow erections to be controlled by the patients. This is sometimes used in younger patients with erectile dysfunction due to organic causes.

Further reading

Tracy JA, Dyck PJ (2008). The spectrum of diabetic neuropathies. *Physical Medicine & Rehabilitation Clinics of North America* **19**, 1–26.

Unger J, Cole BE (2007). Recognition and management of diabetic neuropathy. *Primary Care* **34**, 887–913.

CHAPTER 17

Psychological Issues Related to Diabetes Care

Tim Holt[1] and Sudhesh Kumar[2]

[1]Nuffield Department of Primary Care Health Sciences, Oxford University, UK
[2]Warwick Medical School, University of Warwick; and WISDEM, University Hospital, Coventry, UK

OVERVIEW

- Psychological problems are common in people with diabetes, but most can be overcome with support and education.
- Diabetes is commoner in those with chronic mental illness.
- Problems range from those of adjustment to more serious depressive illness and maladaptive coping behaviours.
- Screening for depression using validated assessment tools should be part of routine surveillance.
- Psychological health is key to successful self-management.
- Family cohesion and agreement about management responsibilities improves metabolic control.

Introduction

Earlier chapters have discussed some of the psychological issues that people with diabetes may encounter – issues with which clinicians should be familiar. There may be positive aspects such as self-efficacy, autonomy and empowerment. However, there may also be more negative aspects, such as the 'learned helplessness' that was mentioned in Chapter 11. We discuss these in more detail here, including more serious disorders of psychological adjustment. We first of all cover some of the less serious issues that most patients may encounter to some degree, before considering the serious problems that affect a small minority.

Adjusting behaviourally to the diagnosis

Diabetes may happen to anyone, and it occurs no less commonly in those with pre-existing psychological or psychiatric disorders, some of which may predispose to diabetes. In type 1 patients, usually presenting in childhood, the personality is still in the developmental stage when the need for dietary discipline, frequent self-injection and blood glucose monitoring arise, all potentially disrupting this formative process (Figure 17.1). It is, therefore, not

surprising that adjustment behaviours may become maladaptive and, sometimes, frankly self-destructive. There is some evidence that children with diabetes are more likely to have difficulties with information processing and learning problems, particularly those children with very early diagnosis or history of severe hypoglycaemia. Poor metabolic control is associated with greater risk of a psychological diagnosis, and frequent hospital admissions lead to recurrent school absence, further disrupting education.

However, there is no one 'personality type' typical of type 1 diabetes, and most adjust remarkably well to these potential stresses, given sufficient support from family and their peers, as well as from their health professionals. In fact, empowered type 1 individuals benefit from the fact that their behaviour is still flexible enough to adapt to the new requirements. This is something that older type 2 patients typically find difficult and, in their cases, it is behavioural inertia and inflexibility that are the obstacles to successful management.

Multidisciplinary behavioural interventions involving the family have been shown to improve regimen adherence and glycaemic control in type 1 children (Box 17.1), but such interventions are usually most effective when introduced soon after the diagnosis.

Needle phobia

A reluctance to pierce the skin with a sharp foreign body is, of course, a perfectly natural response in childhood, and it also affects quite a proportion of adults. Education over the safety of injections, the use of short 5 mm or 6 mm needles and a lot of practice overcome this in the majority of patients, young and old. Type 1 individuals, who rapidly become insulin-dependent, usually solve the problem fairly quickly through repeated exposure to the trigger, as there is no alternative. In older type 2 individuals, however, it may become an unspoken reason why insulin therapy is repeatedly deferred, adding to other sources of inertia.

Demonstrating modern insulin injection technique often overcomes needle phobia, along with supportive encouragement. Familiarity with the device and the injection technique on the part

ABC of Diabetes, Seventh Edition. Tim Holt and Sudhesh Kumar.
© 2015 John Wiley & Sons, Ltd. Published 2015 by John Wiley & Sons, Ltd.

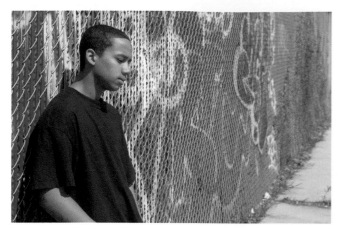

Figure 17.1 Diabetes takes some getting used to even for robust personalities.

Box 17.1 **Components of Effective Behavioural Interventions in Children with Diabetes**

- Goal-setting.
- Self-monitoring.
- Positive reinforcement.
- Behavioural contracts.
- Supportive parental communications.
- Appropriately shared responsibility for diabetes management.

of the clinician is important to foster an atmosphere of confidence-building. If the clinician appears under-confident or clumsy, then this will amplify any anxiety on the patient's side.

A minority of patients remain excessively anxious about insulin injections. Children may become dependent on their parents administering the insulin – a pattern that is, of course, necessary if diabetes occurs in early childhood – but in older children it should be resisted, to promote eventual independence.

'Food addiction'

The pre-existing psychological or psychiatric history of the individual may be very relevant to the patient's adjustment to the diabetes diagnosis and their coping mechanisms. Type 2 diabetes occurs more often in overweight people. Many of these have simply developed bad eating habits in a culture that is increasingly sedentary, and in which high-calorie foods are widely available. Such people may have little or no psychological pathology but, nevertheless, have a serious physical problem that must be overcome by psychological means. A few are obese because of an abnormal attitude towards food and, in some, the term 'food addiction' might be appropriate.

Food addiction has been defined as 'eating types and amounts of foods that seem to contrast with a person's intentions to make moderate and 'sensible' food choices.' However, it is a matter of controversy whether this term is appropriate to people who eat excessively. Nevertheless, those in the severely obese category may benefit from psychological referral in order to explore and address

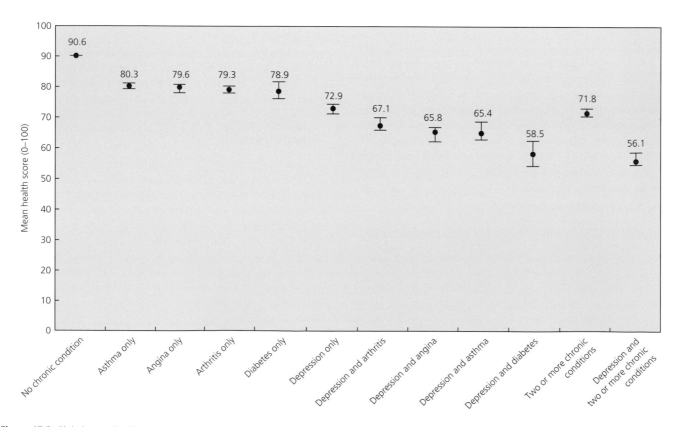

Figure 17.2 Global mean health by disease status. Source: Moussavi *et al.* (2007). Reproduced with permission of Elsevier.

the underlying reasons for their eating behaviour, including body image, the meaning of food in their lives, and their response to hunger and satiety.

Depression and diabetes

While all patients are likely, at times, to feel burdened by the prognostic implications of their diagnosis, a significant proportion will develop potentially serious depressive illnesses. This problem is common enough that it should be actively sought by questioning during regular diabetes reviews, as should some of the issues that

may contribute to it, such as erectile dysfunction. These problems, unlike biochemical indices, are difficult to measure but represent a large component of the person's quality of life.

Depression is a common finding in chronic disease generally, but in the case of diabetes has a particularly significant impact on the mean health score (Figure 17.2).

Depression screening can be undertaken using a validated screening tool involving two questions, following any positive responses with a more detailed questionnaire to assess severity. Three such questionnaires are available. The most commonly used is the PHQ-9 (Table 17.1).

Table 17.1 Patient Health Questionnaire (PHQ-9)

PATIENT, HEALTH QUESTIONNAIRE (PHQ-9)

NAME: _____   DATE: _____

Over the last 2 weeks, how often have you been bothered by any of the following problems?
(*use* "✓" to indicate your answer)

	Not at all	Several days	More than half the days	Nearly every day
1. Little interest or pleasure in doing things			✓	
2. Feeling down, depressed, or hopeless		✓		
3. Trouble falling or staying asleep, or sleeping too much			✓	
4. Feeling tired or having little energy				✓
5. Poor appetite or overeating		✓		
6. Feeling bad about yourself – or that you are a failure or have let yourself or your family down			✓	
7. Trouble concentrating on things, such as reading the newspaper or watching television			✓	
8. Moving or speaking so slowly that other people could having noticed. Or the opposite – being so fidgety or restless that you have been moving around a lot more than usual			✓	
9. Thoughts that you would be better off dead, or of hurting yourself in some way	✓			
add colomns:		2	10	3
TOTAL:			15	

10. If you checked off any problems, how *difficult* have these problems made it for you to do your work, take care of things at home, or get along with other people?	**Not difficult at all** _____ **Somewhat difficult** ✓ _____ **Very difficult** _____ **Extremely difficult** _____

'Self-defeating' behaviour

This psychological condition can affect anyone, with or without diabetes. In the case of the insulin-treated individual, the situation is serious, as the patient has control of a potentially lethal weapon among their self-sabotaging behaviours. It is a pattern that is usually established by early adulthood, and may require intensive psychological treatment, with close liaison between the psychologist and the diabetes team. Behavioural treatments are available, which may involve residential behavioural retraining, but the availability of such programmes is limited.

Milder forms of self-sabotage may occur in many patients, at times of disillusionment or under stressful circumstances. For some people, awaiting a forthcoming diabetes review may be stressful. Such people typically require support to improve their self-efficacy and autonomy.

It is important to distinguish patients who display the more benign forms, or those whose behaviour reflects an underlying depressive illness, from those whose self-defeating behaviour is a more serious primary problem, affecting other areas of their lives, as the treatment approach in each case will be quite different.

Eating disorders in diabetes

We have mentioned above the problem of 'food addiction', in which excessive calorie intake continues way beyond energy requirements, leading to severe obesity and its complications. Diabetes may often be a result, rather than a cause, of this abnormal behaviour.

In addition, people with established anorexia or bulimia nervosa may later develop diabetes, compounding their disordered nutritional status. These problems require co-ordinated, multidisciplinary input from physicians, diabetes nurses, psychiatrists or psychologists and dieticians.

Therapeutic inertia

In the past, reluctance to accept insulin therapy in people with type 2 diabetes was often attributed to patient-centred issues, including their reluctance to engage in a new life pattern of daily or more frequent injections.

More recently, it has been recognised that the problem is compounded through an interaction between patient- and practitioner-centred factors. Recognising our own complicity in this process is important. We may be responsible for amplifying anxiety through our own lack of confidence with managing insulin, or simply by referring to it as if it is a desperate last-resort measure. Similarly, patients and clinicians may vacillate for months over blood pressure treatment or the addition of second or third drugs in the regimen. Patients may pick up signals from the clinician, reinforcing the assumption that the need for medication simply results from failure of lifestyle change. While lifestyle change is effective and should be actively promoted, such an assumption is unfair as the majority will also need medication to achieve ideal targets (Box 17.2).

Summary

Even the most robust personalities will find diabetes a challenge, particularly type 1 patients, who must adapt behaviourally over a short time scale to develop new habits and daily practices, including

---

Box 17.2 **To Avoid Therapeutic Inertia:**

- Mention the range of possible treatments early on, including insulin (using positive language), preferably at one of the early appointments after the diagnosis.
- Discuss the fact that, even if not needed now, insulin is often required at a later stage in type 2 diabetes, as blood glucose levels tend to become more difficult to control.
- Emphasise the benefits of tight blood pressure control in diabetes, mentioning early on that two or three different drug classes are usually required to achieve this.
- It will therefore not be 'their fault' if the patient eventually requires insulin and more than one antihypertensive medication.
- Reassure the patient that there are several different classes, and many different individual antihypertensive drugs, available – it is therefore likely that a suitable combination will be found for them.

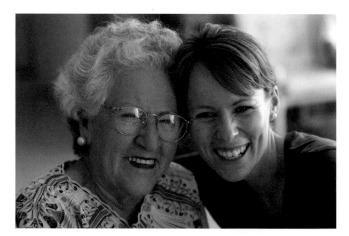

Figure 17.3 With support from family, friends, and health professionals many of the psychological challenges of diabetes can be overcome.

insulin injections. Others may feel the burden of long-term complications, or a fear of them developing in the future. Many simply feel out of control, and it is through addressing this feeling that the greatest impact can be made. The empowered patient who has 'ownership' of their diabetes is likely to have improved quality of life and lower psychological morbidity (Figure 17.3). Health professionals should nurture self-efficacy in all patients, while remaining aware of the possibility of more serious psychological problems. Depression is common in diabetes, and the combination is very detrimental to quality of life. For children with diabetes, behavioural interventions should be family-centred and, preferably, started soon after diagnosis, where the need is evident.

Further reading and references

Delamater AM (2007). Psychological care of children and adolescents with diabetes. *Pediatric Diabetes* **8**, 340–348.

Lloyd CE, Dyer PH, Barnett AH (2000). Prevalence of symptoms of depression and anxiety in a diabetes clinic population. *Diabetic Medicine* **17**, 198–202.

Moussavi S, Chatterji S, Verdes E *et al.* (2007). Depression, chronic disease, and decrements in health: results from the World Health Surveys. *Lancet* **370**, 851–858.

CHAPTER 18

Diabetes and Pregnancy

Sudhesh Kumar[1], Aresh Anwar[2] and Tim Holt[3]

[1]Warwick Medical School, University of Warwick; and WISDEM, University Hospital, Coventry, UK
[2]Royal Perth Hospital, WA, Australia
[3]Nuffield Department of Primary Care Health Sciences, Oxford University, UK

OVERVIEW

- Pregnancy may precipitate diabetes in previously healthy but susceptible individuals.

- Diabetes raises the risk of a complicated pregnancy, increasing both maternal and perinatal mortality and the risk of congenital malformations.

- Pregnancy may cause deterioration of established diabetic complications, and should be avoided in those with poor glycaemic control.

- Tight control of diabetes during pregnancy reduces adverse outcomes substantially.

- Most patients with pre-existing diabetes will require insulin during pregnancy to achieve optimal targets if they are not already using it.

- Management should be coordinated through close liaison and frequent review by the diabetes, obstetric and midwifery teams.

- Follow-up of women with gestational diabetes after pregnancy is important, to exclude persistent hyperglycaemia and because the lifetime risk of type 2 diabetes is high.

Introduction

The standard of obstetric care for women with diabetes has seen dramatic improvements over the past few decades. Several areas however, continue to cause concern. This is reflected by morbidity and mortality in this cohort of individuals, which remains unacceptably high (Table 18.1).

Preconceptual management in women with pre-existing diabetes

Good pregnancy care starts before conception and finishes long after the birth of the baby. This form of proactive approach has been shown to help reduce the risk of some of the complications.

Women who already have diabetes and are of childbearing age, should have pre-pregnancy counselling and optimisation of glycaemic control prior to the pregnancy. A 30-50% decreased risk for congenital anomaly and perinatal mortality per 11 mmol/mol (1%) reduction in periconception HbA1c has been shown in studies from the UK show. All such patients should be managed in joint diabetic pregnancy clinics, where there is input from both diabetes specialist teams and obstetricians with a team of midwives. Diabetic pregnancies are considered high-risk pregnancies (Tables 18.1 and 18.5), and deliveries should be planned in units with appropriate neonatal care facilities.

As congenital malformations remain a major cause of morbidity, it is critical that optimal metabolic control is achieved *before* conception (Table 18.2). Unplanned pregnancies in women with diabetes should be avoided and, therefore, it is important to address contraception in all such women of childbearing age. This will help in planning pregnancy and optimising conditions for the best pregnancy outcome. The increasing prevalence of pre- diabetes and undiagnosed type 2 diabetes outside pregnancy, in women of childbearing age, suggests that guidance regarding routine screening in this group is going to be of increasing importance in the future, so practitioners need to be increasingly vigilant.

In those mothers with evidence of diabetic complications it is important that these are treated optimally prior to pregnancy. Diabetic women planning pregnancy should be helped to achieve optimal glycaemic control, preferably with HbA1c below 6.1% (43 mmol/mol), although this is often difficult to achieve despite intensive insulin therapy management. Women with diabetes are currently advised to take a dose of folic acid that is over ten times higher than that of women who do not have diabetes (i.e. 5 mg/day). If the above conditions are met, the congenital malformation rate is dramatically reduced to nearly that of control population levels (Figure 18.1).

Patients exposed to poor glycaemic control in the first trimester are at risk of congenital malformations, although a more common scenario is for the patient with poor glycaemic control to experience recurrent miscarriages.

ABC of Diabetes, Seventh Edition. Tim Holt and Sudhesh Kumar.
© 2015 John Wiley & Sons, Ltd. Published 2015 by John Wiley & Sons, Ltd.

Those whose HbA1c is greater than 10% (86 mmol/mol) preconceptually should be strongly advised to avoid pregnancy. Otherwise, there is a two- to fourfold increase in the congenital abnormality rate. Abnormalities include spina bifida, congenital heart disease, microcephaly and anencephaly. In women of South Asian origin, in particular, consanguinity is still a major issue and this will, of course, increase the risk of congenital malformations by itself.

Table 18.1 Increased risks for babies of women with diabetes compared to the non-diabetic population.

Stillbirths	4.7 ×
Death of baby in first four weeks	2.6 ×
Major congenital anomaly	2 ×

Table 18.2 Preconception checklist.

Contraception until tight control achieved (<6.1-6.5%)
Folic acid 5 mg per day
Stop teratogenic drugs – ACE inhibitors, Angiotensin II receptor antagonists and statins in particular
Screen for complications – retinal screen, creatinine, ACR, Blood pressure
Check thyroid function and rubella antibodies
Provide some literature – Diabetes UK website and pregnancy guide

Gestational diabetes vs. diabetes in pregnancy

Not all diabetes predates pregnancy, and ensuring there is clarity surrounding the definition of 'gestational diabetes' has been one of the most challenging and controversial areas in the field.

New criteria for classifying and diagnosing hyperglycaemia first detected during pregnancy have recently been accepted by a group of experts convened by the WHO.

Hyperglycaemia (see Table 18.3 for criteria) first detected at any time during pregnancy should be classified as either:

• diabetes mellitus in pregnancy; or
• gestational diabetes mellitus.

The new criteria, whilst recognizing that principles of management between the two groups are similar, aim to draw attention to the fact that there are also some important differences in the approach, including:

• the need for a detailed assessment for the presence of diabetes-related complications at diagnosis of diabetes, especially complications which can affect pregnancy or be aggravated by it, such as retinopathy and renal impairment;
• the need for a more intensive monitoring and treatment of hyperglycaemia, with pharmacotherapy much more likely to be required to control the hyperglycaemia during pregnancy;
• the need for closer follow-up and ongoing monitoring and treatment of women with diabetes following the pregnancy.

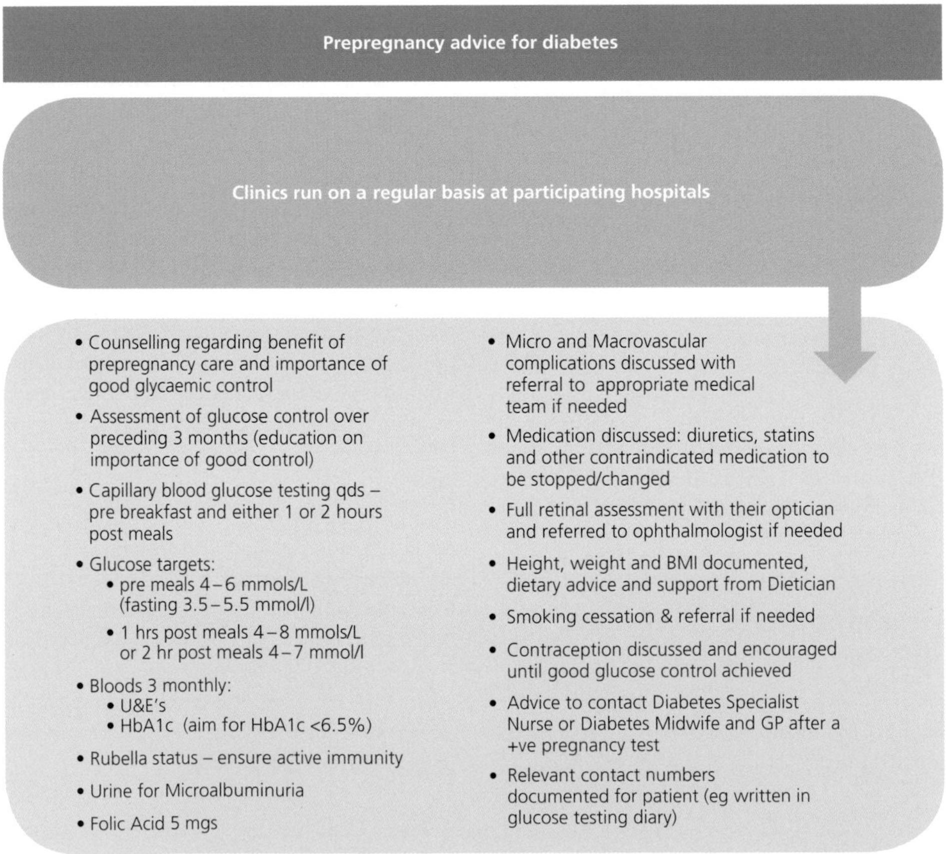

Prepregnancy advice for diabetes

Clinics run on a regular basis at participating hospitals

• Counselling regarding benefit of prepregnancy care and importance of good glycaemic control
• Assessment of glucose control over preceding 3 months (education on importance of good control)
• Capillary blood glucose testing qds – pre breakfast and either 1 or 2 hours post meals
• Glucose targets:
  • pre meals 4–6 mmols/L (fasting 3.5–5.5 mmol/l)
  • 1 hrs post meals 4–8 mmols/L or 2 hr post meals 4–7 mmol/l
• Bloods 3 monthly:
  • U&E's
  • HbA1c (aim for HbA1c <6.5%)
• Rubella status – ensure active immunity
• Urine for Microalbuminuria
• Folic Acid 5 mgs

• Micro and Macrovascular complications discussed with referral to appropriate medical team if needed
• Medication discussed: diuretics, statins and other contraindicated medication to be stopped/changed
• Full retinal assessment with their optician and referred to ophthalmologist if needed
• Height, weight and BMI documented, dietary advice and support from Dietician
• Smoking cessation & referral if needed
• Contraception discussed and encouraged until good glucose control achieved
• Advice to contact Diabetes Specialist Nurse or Diabetes Midwife and GP after a +ve pregnancy test
• Relevant contact numbers documented for patient (eg written in glucose testing diary)

WANDA guidelines No:6. Version 2. Dated Jan 07.

Figure 18.1 Preconceptual advice for women with diabetes planning a pregnancy. Source: Provided by Dr Aresh Anwar.

Screening for 'gestational diabetes'

All pregnant women not known already to have diabetes should have a fasting plasma glucose, HbA1C, or an untimed random plasma glucose at the first antenatal visit. Abnormal results require subsequent confirmation on another day to confirm the diagnosis.

Pregnant women not previously identified before 24 weeks of gestation with diabetes in pregnancy or gestational diabetes should be tested for gestational diabetes (see Table 18.3) by having a two-hour, 75g OGTT performed at 24-28 weeks gestation. Many units use criteria to identify those most at risk in order to define the population to whom they offer a glucose tolerance test (see Box 18.1).

Table 18.3 Classification of diabetes in pregnancy.

Pregnancy in patients with type 1 and type 2 diabetes	Diagnosis of diabetes predates pregnancy
Diabetes mellitus in pregnancy	Diagnosed by the 2006 WHO criteria if one or more of following met: Fasting plasma glucose > 7.0 mmol/l (126 mg/dl) Two-hour plasma glucose > 11.1 mmol/l (200 mg/dl) after 75g GTT Random plasma glucose > 11.1 mmol/l (200 mg/dl) after 75g GTT
Gestational diabetes mellitus (GDM)	GDM diagnosed at any time in pregnancy on any of the following: Fasting plasma glucose = 5.1-6.9 mmol/l (92-125 mg/dl) One-hour post 75 g glucose load hour plasma glucose ≥ 10 mmol/l (180 mg/dl) Two-hour post 75 g glucose load hour plasma glucose 8.5-11.0 mmol/l (153-199 mg/dl) Normally develops in second trimester (24-28 weeks)

Box 18.1 Screening for Gestational Diabetes

At 28 weeks
- First degree relative with diabetes (any type).
- Body mass index >35 kg/m².
- Maternal age >35 years.
- Ethnic minority – South Asian, Afro-Caribbean, Black African.
- Polycystic ovary syndrome.
- Long-term steroids.
- Previous unexplained stillbirth.
- Previous history of macrosomia (birth weight > 4.5 kg or > 90th centile for gestation (on customised growth chart if available)).
- Polyhydramnios or foetal macrosomia in current pregnancy (>90th centile on customised growth chart).

Early screening
Previous history of gestational diabetes should have a glucose tolerance test arranged for 16-20 weeks, with a repeat at 28 weeks if the first is normal.

Immediate screening
Glycosuria ++ or above on two occasions (second sample within 1 week) or +++ on single occasion; urgent blood glucose if significant ketonuria.

Risk factors for screening include obesity, a family history of diabetes, older women and also women in ethnic minorities, particularly South Asians, as it accounts for high rates of gestational diabetes. Those with a history of previous gestational diabetes should be treated as having gestational diabetes during subsequent pregnancies.

Treatment of gestational diabetes

Gestational diabetes is initially treated with diet alone and daily moderate exercise for 30 minutes or more. Options for treatment may include oral hypoglycaemics such as glibenclamide or metformin, but often patients require insulin. In these cases, insulin or the oral hypoglycaemic agents can be stopped upon delivery.

Monitoring of the pregnant patient with diabetes

Organisation of antenatal care and frequency of reviews are summarised in Figure 18.2. HbA1c measures are important pre-conceptually and in the first trimester, but are less useful later in pregnancy, and frequent self-monitoring is required. The patient should visit a joint clinic in the outpatients department, normally every two weeks. Patients are encouraged to check glucose levels post-prandially as well as fasting and pre-prandially, as better control of post-prandial hyperglycaemia can help achieve optimal control (Table 18.4).

Patients with type 2 diabetes who were previously on metformin alone will usually require insulin during pregnancy but, in some cases, especially when they are needle phobic, they are managed safely with glibenclamide, as this does not cross the placental barrier and is not associated with neonatal hypoglycaemia. Metformin has also been shown to be safe in pregnancy, and can be used as a lone agent or with insulin.

The new rapid-acting insulin analogues, such as aspart and lispro, have been found to be particularly useful in pregnancy and to have advantages over soluble insulins. While there is limited data on long-acting analogues, they have slowly become part of routine practice.

Many units, however, continue to advocate the use of isophane in pregnancy. Patients who fail to achieve adequate glycaemic control despite multiple dose regimens should be considered for continuous subcutaneous insulin infusion (an insulin pump).

Managing diabetic complications during pregnancy (see Table 18.5)

Women with pre-existing diabetic retinopathy may experience quite dramatic worsening of this complication with intensifying glycaemic control, especially if they have had poor control before. Therefore, regular examinations are required and they may require laser treatment.

Women with hypertension and/or proteinuria are at great risk of accelerated hypertension and renal failure. In those patients with nephropathy and serum creatinine greater than 200 μmol/l, outcome is likely to be poor. Patients with nephropathy should seek the advice of a nephrologist to discuss their own individual risk before pregnancy. Women with renal impairment can expect some deterioration of renal function following the pregnancy. Hypertension in pregnancy should be managed using methyldopa,

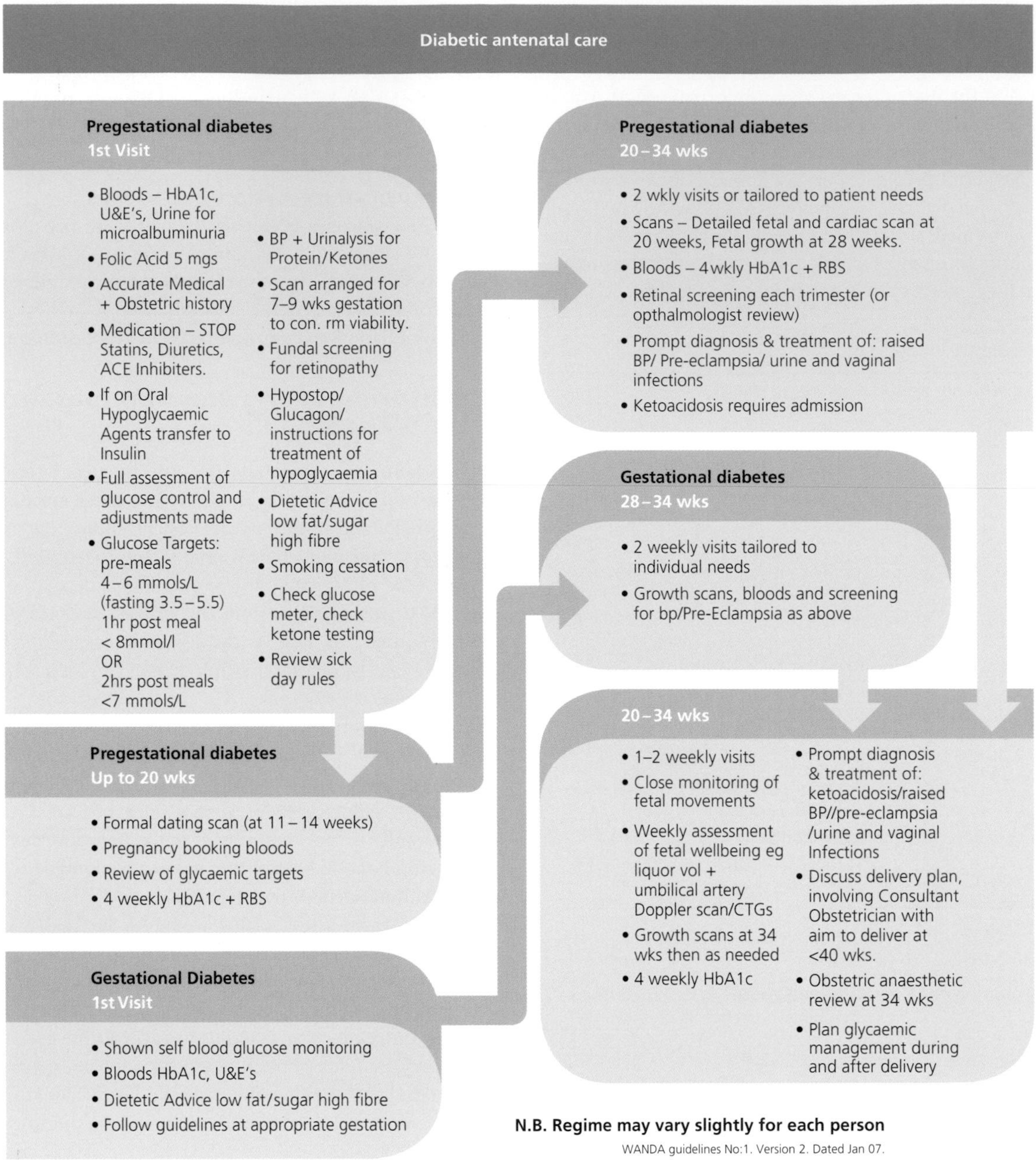

Diabetic antenatal care

Pregestational diabetes
1st Visit

- Bloods – HbA1c, U&E's, Urine for microalbuminuria
- Folic Acid 5 mgs
- Accurate Medical + Obstetric history
- Medication – STOP Statins, Diuretics, ACE Inhibiters.
- If on Oral Hypoglycaemic Agents transfer to Insulin
- Full assessment of glucose control and adjustments made
- Glucose Targets: pre-meals 4–6 mmols/L (fasting 3.5–5.5) 1hr post meal < 8mmol/l OR 2hrs post meals <7 mmols/L

- BP + Urinalysis for Protein/Ketones
- Scan arranged for 7–9 wks gestation to con. rm viability.
- Fundal screening for retinopathy
- Hypostop/ Glucagon/ instructions for treatment of hypoglycaemia
- Dietetic Advice low fat/sugar high fibre
- Smoking cessation
- Check glucose meter, check ketone testing
- Review sick day rules

Pregestational diabetes
Up to 20 wks

- Formal dating scan (at 11–14 weeks)
- Pregnancy booking bloods
- Review of glycaemic targets
- 4 weekly HbA1c + RBS

Gestational Diabetes
1st Visit

- Shown self blood glucose monitoring
- Bloods HbA1c, U&E's
- Dietetic Advice low fat/sugar high fibre
- Follow guidelines at appropriate gestation

Pregestational diabetes
20–34 wks

- 2 wkly visits or tailored to patient needs
- Scans – Detailed fetal and cardiac scan at 20 weeks, Fetal growth at 28 weeks.
- Bloods – 4wkly HbA1c + RBS
- Retinal screening each trimester (or opthalmologist review)
- Prompt diagnosis & treatment of: raised BP/ Pre-eclampsia/ urine and vaginal infections
- Ketoacidosis requires admission

Gestational diabetes
28–34 wks

- 2 weekly visits tailored to individual needs
- Growth scans, bloods and screening for bp/Pre-Eclampsia as above

20–34 wks

- 1–2 weekly visits
- Close monitoring of fetal movements
- Weekly assessment of fetal wellbeing eg liquor vol + umbilical artery Doppler scan/CTGs
- Growth scans at 34 wks then as needed
- 4 weekly HbA1c

- Prompt diagnosis & treatment of: ketoacidosis/raised BP//pre-eclampsia /urine and vaginal Infections
- Discuss delivery plan, involving Consultant Obstetrician with aim to deliver at <40 wks.
- Obstetric anaesthetic review at 34 wks
- Plan glycaemic management during and after delivery

N.B. Regime may vary slightly for each person
WANDA guidelines No:1. Version 2. Dated Jan 07.

Figure 18.2 Organisation of antenatal care for women with diabetes. Source: Provided by Dr Aresh Anwar, University Hospital, Coventry.

Table 18.4 Monitoring targets.

Fasting/pre-meal target	<5.3 mmol/l
Post-prandial target (one hour post meal)	<7.8 mmol/l

together with labetalol or amlodipine, if needed. Those on angiotensin-converting enzyme inhibitors should ideally be changed to the above agents before pregnancy. Statins should be stopped three months prior to planned conception.

Monitoring the foetus during pregnancy

The true value of foetal monitoring continues to be debated. A standard regime will start with a dating scan as soon as possible in pregnancy. This is normally followed by a more accurate dating scan at 11–12 weeks of gestation, and there will then be a detailed scan at 20–21 weeks, specifically examining the foetus for cardiac and central nervous system abnormalities. Serial scans assessing foetal growth normally start at 27 weeks, with units varying the frequency with which they scan patients. A major risk to the foetus from diabetes is macrosomia (21% > 4000 g versus 11% in general population) and a twofold increase in shoulder dystocia (7.9% versus around 3%). Assessment of foetal size, weight and health are important in determining the timing and mode of delivery.

There remains a high risk of unexplained late intrauterine death. The risk of this increases as the pregnancy progresses. As a consequence, pregnancies of patients with diabetes are rarely allowed to progress to full term, and patients are assessed for an appropriate delivery date from 38 weeks. Growth retardation is serious and requires specialist investigation.

Table 18.5 Inter-relationship of diabetes and pregnancy.

Impact of diabetes on the baby
Increased miscarriage rate
Increased risk of congenital anomalies
Increased risk of macrosomia
Increased risk of stillbirth
Increased perinatal mortality

Impact of pregnancy on diabetes
Progression of retinopathy
Progression of nephropathy
Progression of neuropathy

Impact of diabetes on pregnancy
Increased risk of pre-eclampsia
Increased risk of polyhydramnios
Increased risk of Caesarean section

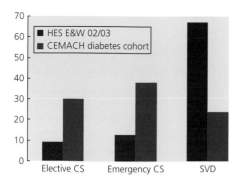

Figure 18.3 Proportion of pregnancies resulting in elective and emergency Caesarean sections (CS) and spontaneous vaginal delivery (SVD), based on Hospital Episode Statistics (HES) for England and Wales (2002/3) and the Confidential Enquiry into Maternal and Child Health (CEMACH) diabetes cohort.

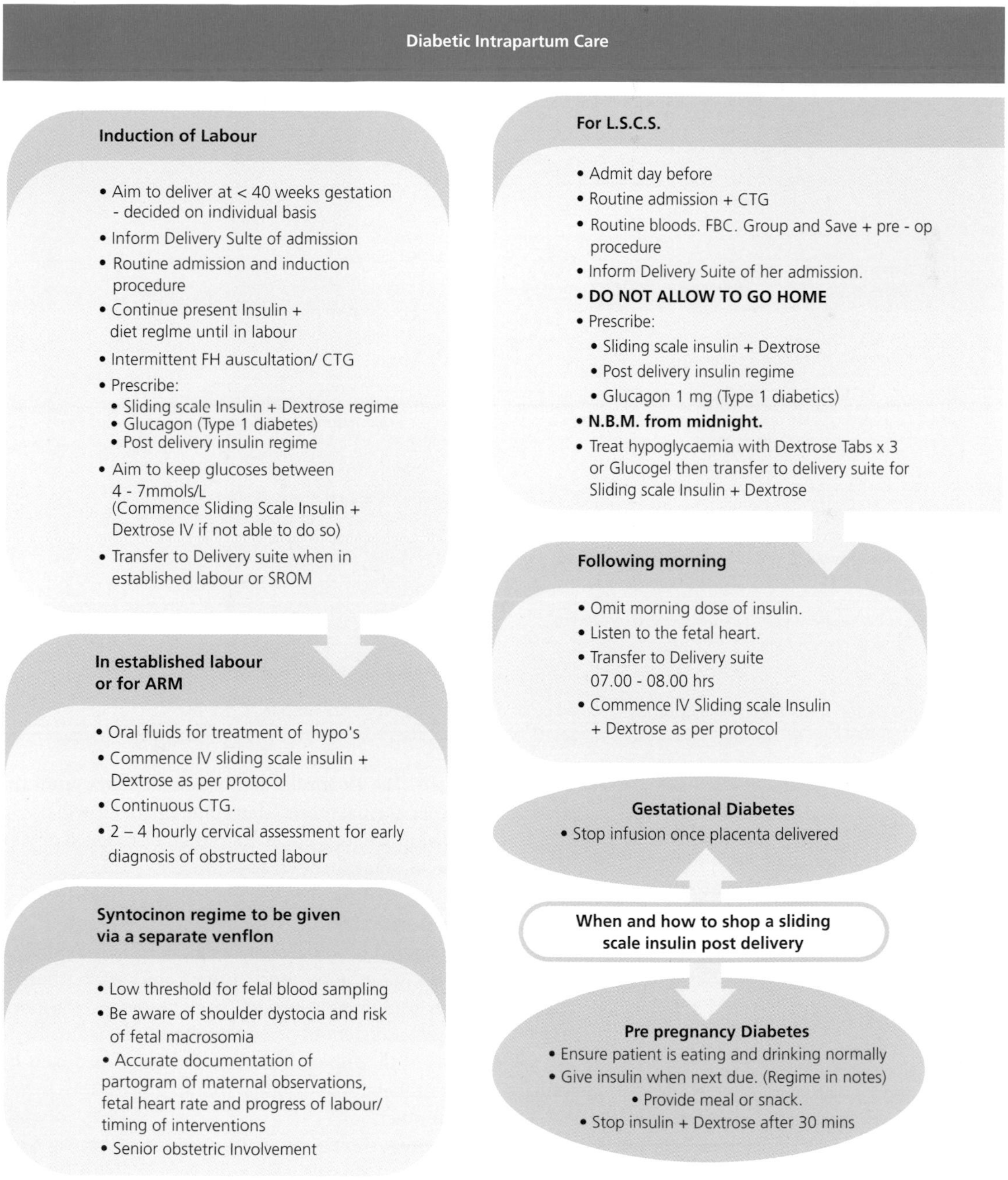

Diabetic Intrapartum Care

Induction of Labour

- Aim to deliver at < 40 weeks gestation - decided on individual basis
- Inform Delivery Suite of admission
- Routine admission and induction procedure
- Continue present Insulin + diet reglme until in labour
- Intermittent FH auscultation/ CTG
- Prescribe:
  - Sliding scale Insulin + Dextrose regime
  - Glucagon (Type 1 diabetes)
  - Post delivery insulin regime
- Aim to keep glucoses between 4 - 7mmols/L (Commence Sliding Scale Insulin + Dextrose IV if not able to do so)
- Transfer to Delivery suite when in established labour or SROM

In established labour or for ARM

- Oral fluids for treatment of hypo's
- Commence IV sliding scale insulin + Dextrose as per protocol
- Continuous CTG.
- 2 – 4 hourly cervical assessment for early diagnosis of obstructed labour

Syntocinon regime to be given via a separate venflon

- Low threshold for felal blood sampling
- Be aware of shoulder dystocia and risk of fetal macrosomia
- Accurate documentation of partogram of maternal observations, fetal heart rate and progress of labour/ timing of interventions
- Senior obstetric Involvement

For L.S.C.S.

- Admit day before
- Routine admission + CTG
- Routine bloods. FBC. Group and Save + pre - op procedure
- Inform Delivery Suite of her admission.
- **DO NOT ALLOW TO GO HOME**
- Prescribe:
  - Sliding scale insulin + Dextrose
  - Post delivery insulin regime
  - Glucagon 1 mg (Type 1 diabetics)
- **N.B.M. from midnight.**
- Treat hypoglycaemia with Dextrose Tabs x 3 or Glucogel then transfer to delivery suite for Sliding scale Insulin + Dextrose

Following morning

- Omit morning dose of insulin.
- Listen to the fetal heart.
- Transfer to Delivery suite 07.00 - 08.00 hrs
- Commence IV Sliding scale Insulin + Dextrose as per protocol

Gestational Diabetes
- Stop infusion once placenta delivered

When and how to shop a sliding scale insulin post delivery

Pre pregnancy Diabetes
- Ensure patient is eating and drinking normally
- Give insulin when next due. (Regime in notes)
- Provide meal or snack.
- Stop insulin + Dextrose after 30 mins

N.B. Regime may vary slightly for each person, please check notes

WANDA. guidelines No:2. Version 2. Dated Jan 07.

Figure 18.4 Management of blood glucose during delivery. Source: Provided by Dr Aresh Anwar, University Hospital, Coventry.

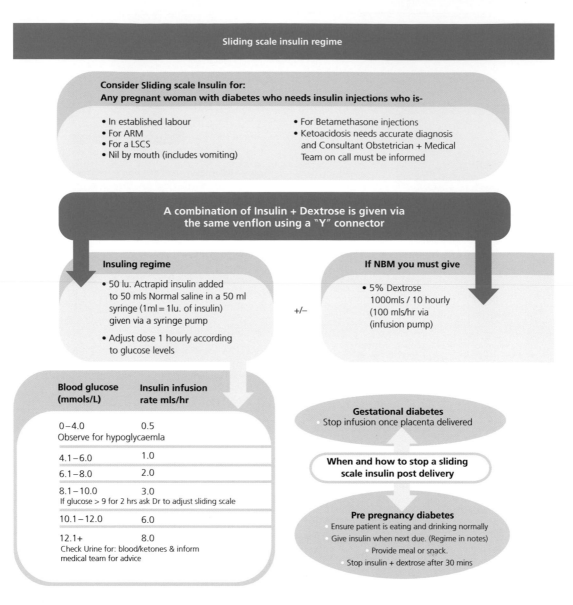

Sliding scale insulin regime

Consider Sliding scale Insulin for:
Any pregnant woman with diabetes who needs insulin injections who is-

- In established labour
- For ARM
- For a LSCS
- Nil by mouth (includes vomiting)

- For Betamethasone injections
- Ketoacidosis needs accurate diagnosis and Consultant Obstetrician + Medical Team on call must be informed

A combination of Insulin + Dextrose is given via the same venflon using a "Y" connector

Insuling regime

- 50 lu. Actrapid insulin added to 50 mls Normal saline in a 50 ml syringe (1ml = 1lu. of insulin) given via a syringe pump
- Adjust dose 1 hourly according to glucose levels

+/−

If NBM you must give

- 5% Dextrose 1000mls / 10 hourly (100 mls/hr via (infusion pump)

Blood glucose (mmols/L)	Insulin infusion rate mls/hr
0–4.0 Observe for hypoglycaemla	0.5
4.1–6.0	1.0
6.1–8.0	2.0
8.1–10.0 If glucose > 9 for 2 hrs ask Dr to adjust sliding scale	3.0
10.1–12.0	6.0
12.1+ Check Urine for: blood/ketones & inform medical team for advice	8.0

Gestational diabetes
- Stop infusion once placenta delivered

When and how to stop a sliding scale insulin post delivery

Pre pregnancy diabetes
- Ensure patient is eating and drinking normally
- Give insulin when next due. (Regime in notes)
- Provide meal or snack.
- Stop insulin + dextrose after 30 mins

WANDA guidelines No:4. Version 2. Dated Jan 07.

Figure 18.5 Insulin sliding scale for use during delivery. Source: Provided by Dr Aresh Anwar, University Hospital, Coventry.

Management in labour

Pregnant women with diabetes are usually admitted for a short period before the planned delivery, or for a longer period when there are complications present. Monitoring of hyperglycaemia and also of the foetal heart rate is carried out. Although the aim is for a vaginal delivery in most cases, it is still by Caesarean section in many cases, at around 38 weeks gestation (Figure 18.3).

Managing hyperglycaemia during labour

All obstetric units will have a regime for managing hyperglycaemia during labour. An example is given in Figures 18.4 and 18.5. Glucose and insulin are given by IV infusion, and the rate of insulin infusion is adjusted to maintain blood glucose levels between 4-7

mmol/l. The IV insulin pump is maintained until the mother can start her normal meals. Many type 2 patients will not require insulin following delivery, but doses should be reduced or adjusted according to plasma glucose levels.

The neonate

The most common neonatal complication is hypoglycaemia, which still occurs in about one in five babies of mothers with diabetes. Hyperinsulinaemia results from placental transport of maternal insulin (endogenous or administered) that is surplus to the requirements of the infant. This is the cause of neonatal hypoglycaemia (and of foetal macrosomia, due to growth in a hyperinsulinaemic environment).

Feeding should be encouraged as soon as possible (within 30 minutes) after delivery and every 2-3 hours thereafter. Neonatal

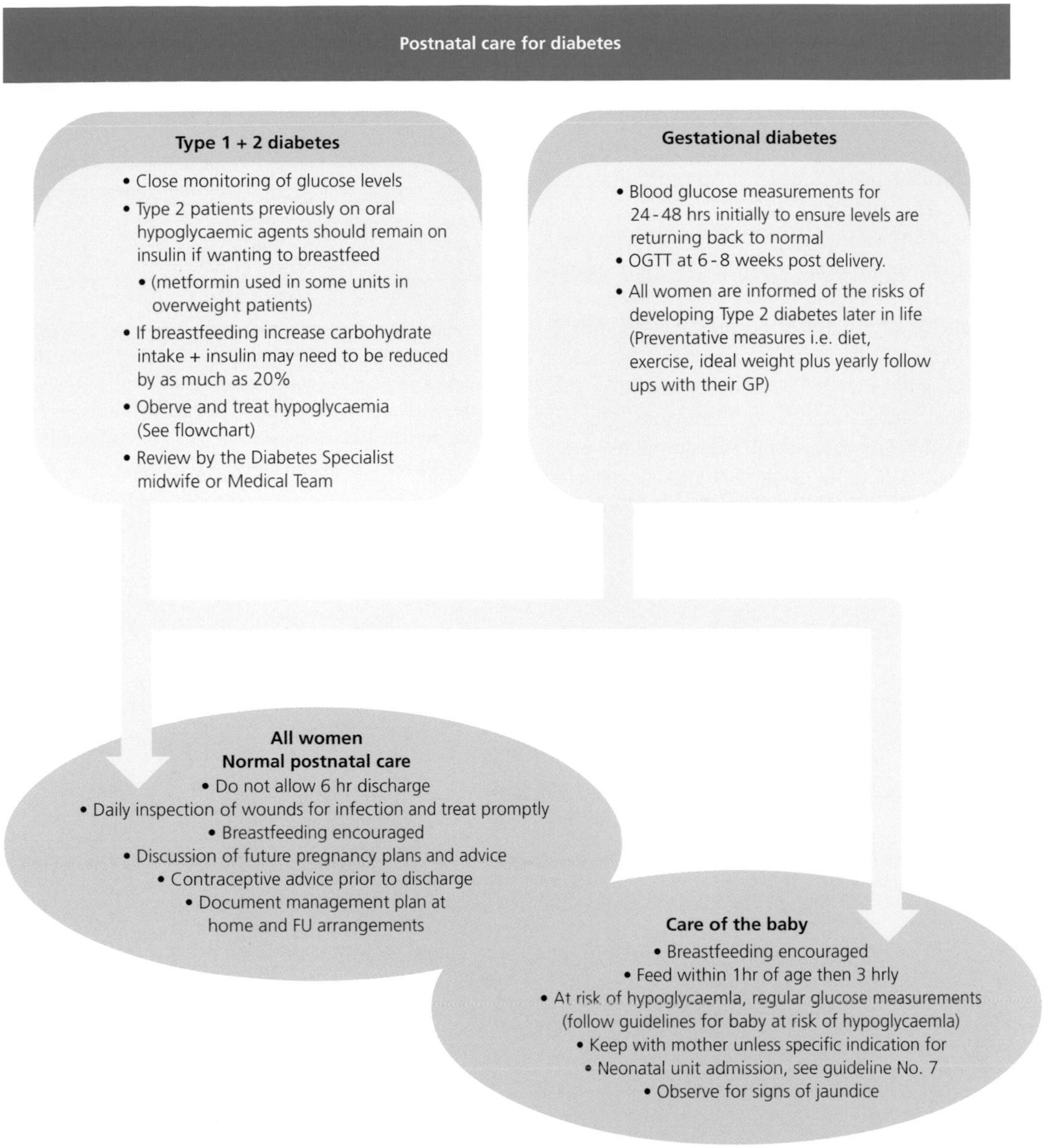

Postnatal care for diabetes

Type 1 + 2 diabetes

- Close monitoring of glucose levels
- Type 2 patients previously on oral hypoglycaemic agents should remain on insulin if wanting to breastfeed
  - (metformin used in some units in overweight patients)
- If breastfeeding increase carbohydrate intake + insulin may need to be reduced by as much as 20%
- Oberve and treat hypoglycaemia (See flowchart)
- Review by the Diabetes Specialist midwife or Medical Team

Gestational diabetes

- Blood glucose measurements for 24-48 hrs initially to ensure levels are returning back to normal
- OGTT at 6-8 weeks post delivery.
- All women are informed of the risks of developing Type 2 diabetes later in life (Preventative measures i.e. diet, exercise, ideal weight plus yearly follow ups with their GP)

All women
Normal postnatal care
- Do not allow 6 hr discharge
- Daily inspection of wounds for infection and treat promptly
- Breastfeeding encouraged
- Discussion of future pregnancy plans and advice
- Contraceptive advice prior to discharge
- Document management plan at home and FU arrangements

Care of the baby
- Breastfeeding encouraged
- Feed within 1hr of age then 3 hrly
- At risk of hypoglycaemla, regular glucose measurements (follow guidelines for baby at risk of hypoglycaemla)
- Keep with mother unless specific indication for
- Neonatal unit admission, see guideline No. 7
- Observe for signs of jaundice

WANDA guidelines No:5. Version 2. Dated Jan 07.

Figure 18.6 Postnatal care guidelines for all types of diabetes in pregnancy. Source: Provided by Dr Aresh Anwar, University Hospital, Coventry.

blood glucose levels should be monitored regularly. If the level remains below 2.0 mmol/l on two occasions, despite adequate feeding (or if feeding is ineffective), then tube-feeding or intravenous dextrose should be considered. Respiratory distress syndrome is a complication if the baby is delivered prematurely, particularly when the mother has had poor glycaemic control. Occasionally, other complications, such as polycythaemia and hypocalcaemia may occur. Macrosomia contributes significantly both to maternal and neonatal morbidity.

Breastfeeding is encouraged just as in non-diabetic mothers, and the mother's diet is increased by about 50 g of carbohydrate daily. Breastfeeding mothers should not use oral hypoglycaemic agents. The use of metformin during breastfeeding is not recommended by the manufacturers.

Postnatal follow-up of gestational diabetes

Following the postnatal checks, a glucose tolerance test is arranged about 6–8 weeks after delivery. A majority of patients return to normal glucose tolerance; however, these women do have an increased risk of developing type 2 diabetes over the next five years. Even if the glucose tolerance test is normal, an annual check of fasting blood glucose is advised, and they are advised to continue with a healthy lifestyle. They should also be told that they are virtually certain to have gestational diabetes in future pregnancies.

Those diagnosed to have persistent diabetes following the postnatal glucose tolerance test are treated like other patients with type 2 diabetes. Figure 18.6 summarises postpartum care for mothers and babies, following a diabetic pregnancy.

Summary

Pregnancy places a physiological strain on maternal glucose tolerance, precipitating gestational diabetes in those at risk and threatening to destabilise pre-existing diabetes. In either scenario, a substantially increased risk of complicated pregnancy justifies proactive, coordinated management in order to improve maternal and neonatal outcomes. This approach should commence before pregnancy through preconceptual interventions, including tightening of glycaemic control, withdrawal of potentially teratogenic medications and prescription of high dose folic acid.

The majority of patients affected will require insulin during pregnancy to achieve optimal glycaemic targets, and the newer rapid-acting insulin analogues may be particularly useful in this setting. Delivery of the infant may restore previous glucose tolerance in the mother, but close monitoring is required to detect neonatal hypoglycaemia. For those with gestational diabetes diagnosed during the pregnancy, follow-up is essential to confirm resolution and to screen for future incident diabetes. Patient education is important at all stages to optimise outcomes.

Further reading

Diagnostic Criteria and Classification of Hyperglycaemia First Detected in Pregnancy. World Health Organization, Geneva, August 2013.

Confidential Enquiry into Maternal and Child Health (CEMACH) (2005). *Pregnancy in Women with Type 1 and Type 2 Diabetes in 2002-03, England, Wales and Northern Ireland.* London, CEMACH.

Getahun D, Nath C, Ananth CV *et al.* (2008). Gestational diabetes in the United States: temporal trends 1989 through 2004. *American Journal of Obstetrics & Gynecology* **198**(5), 525.e1–5.

National Institute of Health and Clinical Excellence (2008). *Diabetes in pregnancy.* Clinical guideline No 63.

Guideline Development Group, NICE and Mugglestone M (2008). Management of diabetes from preconception to the postnatal period: summary of NICE guidance. *BMJ* **336**(7646), 714–717.

Zhang X, Decker A, Platt RW, Kramer MS (2008). How big is too big? The perinatal consequences of fetal macrosomia. *American Journal of Obstetrics & Gynecology* **198**(5), 517.e1–6.

CHAPTER 19

Organisation of Diabetes Care in General Practice

Tim Holt[1] and Sudhesh Kumar[2]

[1]Nuffield Department of Primary Care Health Sciences, Oxford University, UK
[2]Warwick Medical School, University of Warwick; and WISDEM, University Hospital, Coventry, UK

OVERVIEW

- Quality diabetes care requires well-developed organisational infrastructure.

- The Diabetes Register is central both for surveillance and audit.

- Annual reviews should be offered to all patients, but most will require more frequent contact to monitor progress towards targets, address emerging problems and screen for early complications.

- Monitoring quality of care may be a practice-based activity, or it may occur at a higher level through integrated information technology, depending on the healthcare setting.

- Measuring quality of care should include not only numerical indices that are electronically coded but also the qualitative aspects, including access, continuity and patient satisfaction.

Introduction

The majority of diabetes care, particularly for type 2 patients, can be provided by non-specialist clinicians who have ready access to specialist advice. The increasing prevalence of type 2 diabetes makes this the most effective use of resources, saving specialist expertise for when it is really required. Primary care clinicians need to maintain and develop their expertise within a multidisciplinary team of professionals. Structured care programmes, involving regular surveillance, and clearly understood referral pathways to secondary care, are essential components of this infrastructure.

Diabetes Register

Central to any surveillance programme is the Diabetes Register. Ideally, everyone with diabetes should be recorded on the Diabetes Register of one care provider. This provider can then identify all the patients with diabetes for whom the team is responsible. In this way, it is clear to everyone who is responsible for whose care. In the UK, this is achieved through registration in general practice, and all NHS patients have a NHS number that is their 'unique identifier'.

The general practitioners manage the majority of diabetes surveillance and, for patients under hospital follow-up (including most children), they can audit the control parameters as a back-up to hospital-based audits. This means that the primary care diabetes registers include everyone known to have diabetes in the community.

> While patients increasingly take and share responsibility for treatment decisions and follow up, health care providers must recognise their own corporate responsibility for ensuring high-quality care to all their registered patients.

Quality of the Diabetes Register

Organisation of care revolves around the register, but we should not forget about those in the community who are missing from it (see the overlapping but non-identical circles in Figure 19.1). No diabetes register is perfect, and it is likely to not only miss a significant number of cases (estimated 850,000 in the UK) but also to include patients who on more rigorous testing would not fulfil the diagnostic criteria. Mechanisms for improving and maintaining the quality of the diabetes register should be built into the daily processes of routine care, to ensure as close an overlap as possible. These include active case finding for undiagnosed patients, adherence to recommended criteria for diagnosis, and removal of patients from the register that have moved out of the area and registered for care elsewhere.

In most economically developed countries, the Register will take the form of an electronic database. However, whatever form it takes, two requirements are essential:

- The Register can identify everyone known to have diabetes.
- Searches can be undertaken to identify individuals who are due surveillance or whose results are out of target.

In the UK, surveillance for complications takes place predominantly in primary care. Chapter 12 describes the regular surveillance procedures recommended as part of structured care (Boxes 19.1 and 19.2).

ABC of Diabetes, Seventh Edition. Tim Holt and Sudhesh Kumar.

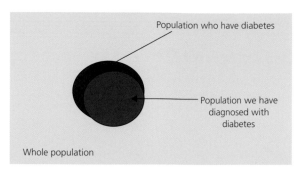

Figure 19.1 A high quality diabetes register ensures the population with diabetes is identified as accurately as possible so that the circles overlap closely.

Box 19.1 **Overall Aim of Diabetes Care**

- To achieve a quality of life and life expectancy similar to that of the general population
- To reduce the symptoms and the complications of diabetes whilst enjoying a flexible life-style
- To treat those with diabetes individually and involve them in all aspects of their care, empowering them with the knowledge and skills to feel in control of their diabetes

Box 19.2 **Cornerstones of Diabetes Care Organisation**

- Identification of those at risk
- Reduction of both diabetes and cardiovascular risk in the 'at-risk' population
- Early detection of diabetes
- Comprehensive education and life-style advice tailored to the individual and carers
- Prescribed medication and referral within an extended team of professionals
- Access to information and help during and between regular reviews
- Regular surveillance for complications
- Early, active intervention for developing complications

Case finding for diabetes

Screening the whole population for diabetes is inefficient and not currently recommended, but *case finding* by targeting at-risk groups (Box 19.3) is worthwhile.

How often should we test?

Generally speaking, at least every three years. However, people with impaired glucose tolerance (IGT), impaired fasting glycaemia (IFG) or a history of gestational diabetes require testing annually (see below), and should be advised to return sooner if diabetes symptoms develop in the meantime.

Box 19.3 **Groups who Justify Regular Testing for Diabetes**

- Known cardiovascular disease, hypertension or hyperlipidaemia.
- Impaired glucose tolerance or impaired fasting glycaemia.
- Metabolic syndrome characteristics.
- Family history of type 2 diabetes.
- Ethnicity: South Asian, Afro-Caribbean, American Indian, Pacific Islanders.
- History of gestational diabetes.
- Drug therapy (e.g. corticosteroids).
- Polycystic ovaries plus obesity.
- Chronic mental illness.

Follow-up of borderline random blood glucose results

Random glucose measurements equal to or above 6.1 justify follow-up testing by fasting plasma glucose (FPG) and HbA1c. Before arranging this, find out:

1 Does the patient have any symptoms of diabetes (thirst, polyuria, unexplained weight loss)?
2 Was the original blood glucose test actually random or fasting (this may be unclear in the notes)?

Diabetes needs then to be established or excluded in the way described in Chapter 1. Clinical suspicion of diabetes may justify repeated testing at intervals determined by perceived risk.

Follow-up of gestational diabetes

Those with a history of gestational diabetes are at raised life-long risk of type 2 diabetes. Where glucose tolerance has returned to normal after delivery, a fasting plasma glucose should be offered annually.

Organising care following the diagnosis

Explaining the diagnosis to the patient

The quality of explanation and information given to the newly diagnosed patient is an important factor in long-term concordance and in promoting self-efficacy, and so is worth the time investment. Patients sometimes have specific beliefs about the cause of diabetes or why it has happened to them. These are worth discussing. From an organisational point of view, the time required to cover these areas needs protecting.

Initial assessment

Measurements. At the first assessment following the diagnosis, the following measurements should be taken:

- Weight
- Body mass index
- Height
- Waist circumference
- Blood pressure
- Urine for microalbumin

Monitoring and surveillance arrangements

- Arrange retinopathy screening.
- Arrange blood test for:
  - baseline HbA1c (unless already done in the past three months);
  - urea and electrolytes and estimated glomerular filtration rate (e-GFR);
  - liver function tests;
  - baseline fasting lipids, including total serum cholesterol, HDL cholesterol, LDL cholesterol and triglycerides.

The majority of patients presenting will have type 2 diabetes, and be at least overweight at diagnosis. If the patient has a normal body mass index, or is losing weight, this should be noted and drawn to the attention of a clinician responsible for insulin initiation. Such patients may be insulin-deficient and might need insulin early on in the course of their treatment.

Treatment pathways are discussed in Chapters 7 and 9, and surveillance in Chapter 11.

Follow-up

After the initial assessment, a follow-up appointment should be made at an appropriate interval. For most type 2 patients, treatment decisions will need to be reviewed after 2-3 months. Regular reviews during this period are a good idea to answer questions, build confidence, reinforce successful changes and detect the occasional patient with deteriorating insulin deficiency. Generally, type 2 patients out of target for HbA1c should be reviewed with repeat HbA1c every three months after each change in treatment until in target, then six-monthly thereafter.

Starting insulin in general practice

Type 1 patients who present acutely should be referred without delay to secondary care services. They may or may not need hospital admission, but are at risk of ketoacidosis and require close monitoring, education and frequent follow-up in the early stages. This is best carried out under the supervision of a specialist team, including diabetes specialist nurses. The management of type 2 patients requiring insulin is discussed in Chapters 7 and 9.

Assessing the quality of diabetes care

The Quality and Outcomes Framework

One of the advantages of a searchable diabetes register is the ease with which regular audit on the quality of care may be carried out. In the United Kingdom, this facility is provided through the 'Quality and Outcomes Framework', introduced in April 2004 (Figure 19.2). General practitioners are given payments according to the proportion of patients achieving specified quality standards at the end of the year.

Each audit standard attracts payment 'points', whose value relates to the importance of the parameter as a determinant of outcomes and its achievability. Regular practice meetings identify areas of care that are falling short of the standards specified. The patients currently out of target for each parameter can be readily identified through a drop-down box accessed by clicking on the appropriate page. A system of alert messages identifies which parameters are out of target each time a patient's notes are opened. The QOF relies on a system of integrated practice-based software, linked to the local laboratory, and on the consistent electronic coding of the necessary parameters.

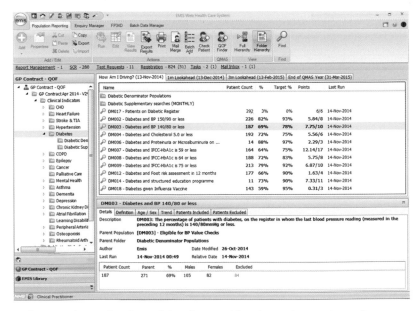

Figure 19.2 Population manager software at the practice of one of the editors, enabling the practice team to monitor progress towards treatment targets and listing the 'points' available for each indicator. The annual influenza immunisation programme is yet to start. Work is required on the proportion of patients with albuminuria who are prescribed ACE inhibitors or A2RB agents (currently only 76% against a target of 80%). Individuals outside any of the targets are easily identifiable through drop-down lists, and their medical records can then be browsed directly. Other UK-based clinical software systems provide similar facilities. Source: EMIS.

Box 19.4 Cases Worth Examining and Discussing Among the Team

- **A type 2 patient presenting with HbA1c > 108 mmol/mol at diagnosis**. This suggests late presentation (unless the clinical picture is that of insulin deficiency, with weight loss). Looking back through the records over five years, were previous borderline or raised blood glucose levels recorded but not followed up? Were possible diabetes symptoms reported but not investigated with diabetes in mind? Was the patient identifiably at risk but not included in active case finding?
- **A patient requiring amputation**. This is a serious event that may reflect a failure of preventive care. Was everything done to minimise the risk of this complication? Was the protocol for surveillance followed, and is it understood by the entire team? Were risk factors identified and actively managed? Are the indications and mechanisms for referral to secondary care widely understood within the practice?
- **A patient not requesting important medication**. Are the practice's mechanisms for access to repeat prescriptions and consultations robust? Are there difficulties in accessing help? Does the patient understand the importance of regular review? If not, why not?

Payment by results: pros and cons

The benefits for patient care resulting from the QOF are evident using intermediate outcome measures such as blood pressure and glycaemic control. It will take longer to demonstrate an impact on mortality and serious morbidity. Many in primary care welcome the QOF and, in the main, general practitioners feel they are being paid appropriately for the evidence-based management of serious chronic disease, while patient advocacy groups recognise the potential benefits arising from financial incentives.

However, there are negative aspects. There may be adverse effects on clinician-patient relationships due to primary care having become extremely target-driven, and the aspects of care that are not easily measured may be out-prioritised. Clinicians may become preoccupied with numerical data and neglect the qualitative aspects of care that patients value. Another criticism is that the same targets are applied to heterogeneous sub-groups of patients, failing to recognise individual needs, and that the elderly may be treated too aggressively. The QOF is reviewed annually to examine such effects, and changes are made based on wide consultation with stakeholding bodies, including those that represent patients and their carers.

Significant events

Care may be improved by team discussion of 'significant events', where issues or problems have arisen that might have been dealt with better. This should be a regular activity. It is based on individual cases, and should supplement (not simply replace) a regular programme of audit involving the entire population with diabetes under the team's care. Possible significant events that may be worth examining are suggested in Box 19.4, but there are many other possibilities.

Patient satisfaction and feedback

Patients should be offered opportunities to feed back and comment on the quality of care provided by the team. This should involve both active and passive strategies:

- Patient satisfaction surveys, carried out periodically, to seek feedback actively.
- Suggestions box.
- Complaints procedure.
- Patient support groups feeding back to the practice team.

Summary

Well-developed organisational infrastructure is essential to high-quality diabetes care. Multidisciplinary teamwork requires clearly understood processes and referral pathways, providing good communication and clear allocation of clinical and administrative responsibilities. These processes should cover:

- the early detection and diagnosis of diabetes, through which individuals enter the diabetes register;
- the initial assessment and education of the patient;
- regular surveillance, follow-up and cross-referral within the extended team; and
- availability of interventions for the effective prevention and treatment of complications.

Further reading

Morris AD, Boyle DIR, MacAlpine R, *et al.* (1997). The diabetes audit and research in Tayside Scotland (DARTS) study: electronic record linkage to create a diabetes register. *BMJ* **315**, 524–528.

Evans JMM, Newton RW, Ruta DA, MacDonald TM, Stevenson RJ, Morris AD (1999). Frequency of blood glucose monitoring in relation to glycaemic control: observational study with diabetes database. *BMJ* **319**, 83–86.

The Quality and Outcomes Framework (QOF): http://www.qof.ic.nhs.uk/

CHAPTER 20

New and Emerging Therapies for Diabetes

Tim Holt[1] and Sudhesh Kumar[2]

[1]Nuffield Department of Primary Care Health Sciences, Oxford University, UK
[2]Warwick Medical School, University of Warwick; and WISDEM, University Hospital, Coventry, UK

OVERVIEW

- Modern management of both hyperglycaemia and obesity is still inadequate for a substantial proportion of patients.

- Progressive beta cell failure is particularly difficult to treat in overweight patients who are insulin-resistant.

- Emerging approaches involve new physiological pathways, including the incretin system and the SLGT2 inhibitors that produce renal glycosuria.

- Future progress is likely to involve not only novel drug classes but also non-pharmacological approaches, including islet cell transplantation and the artificial pancreas.

Introduction

Despite the best efforts of the patient and supporting clinicians, it is not always possible to control diabetes adequately, prevent the progression of the condition or treat its devastating complications. Part of the problem may be related to the heterogeneity of diabetes that we currently ignore in our empirical approach to the management of hyperglycaemia. In the future, personalised therapy based, on the underlying causes, may help to improve outcomes. The last few years have seen intense activity in the pharmaceutical and biotechnology industries to develop more varied modalities of treatment for controlling hyperglycaemia.

Key limitations of current therapeutic approaches

There are a number of barriers to effective control of hyperglycaemia associated with current therapy. First, it should be recognised that major limitations exist in our delivery of diabetes care and in empowering patients to self-manage their condition. Improvements here will help in getting better outcomes from our existing therapies. Some features of type 2 diabetes, in particular, make it difficult to manage with our existing therapies. The most important problems are:

- **Beta cell failure.** Prevention of beta cell destruction could potentially prevent type 1 diabetes in susceptible individuals, and significantly reduce the risk of progression of type 2 diabetes and the need for insulin.
- **Obesity.** One problem with a number of our therapies for diabetes is weight gain. This is not appreciated by patients, and with obesity comes many other risk factors because of the known relationship between obesity, blood pressure and dyslipidaemia.
- **Hypoglycaemia.** This is a feared complication of diabetes and a major impediment to improving glycaemic control. Hypoglycaemia can blight an individual's life, and it is important to try and avoid this.
- **Insulin resistance.** Type 2 diabetes is, in part, due to defects in insulin action. In those with marked insulin defects, this means large doses of insulin and difficulty in achieving tight glucose control.
- **Control of post-prandial hyperglycaemia.** Recently, there has been more attention given to post-prandial hyperglycaemia, because of recognition of its relationship to vascular disease risk. Control of post-prandial hyperglycaemia is important in order to get better control of overall hyperglycaemia.
- **Side-effects of medication.** There are side-effects related to various drugs available today that limit therapy, for example gastrointestinal side effects with metformin and alpha-glycosidase inhibitors, fluid retention and osteopaenia with thiazolidinediones (glitazones) and hypoglycaemia and weight gain for sulphonylureas. Indeed, the use of thiazolidinediones has declined substantially because of the side-effect profile.

Many of the following groups of newer drugs are advantageous in terms of one or more of the above aspects. However, one limitation of newer therapies is that we do not yet have evidence of long-term benefits through reduction of complications or long-term safety. Therefore, the potential for improvement in hyperglycaemia and lack of side-effects must be placed in the above context.

ABC of Diabetes, Seventh Edition. Tim Holt and Sudhesh Kumar.
© 2015 John Wiley & Sons, Ltd. Published 2015 by John Wiley & Sons, Ltd.

Pramlintide

Pramlintide is an antidiabetic agent that mimics the activity of the hormone amylin, which is co-secreted along with insulin from the pancreatic islets. It is available in the United States for mealtime control of hyperglycaemia, as an addition to insulin therapy. It acts mainly by altering the rate of gastric emptying, and also by reducing the rise of glucagon levels following meals. It is given as a separate injection to insulin and can produce additional improvement in glucose control. It is currently not available in the UK.

Incretins and other hormone-based therapies

Incretins are endogenous gut hormones, including glucagon-like peptide-1 (GLP-1) and glucose-dependant insulinotrophic polypeptide (GIP). They have useful insulin-releasing and other glucose-regulatory actions. Preparations of GLP-1 analogues, or modified formulations of this peptide (GLP-1 mimetics), have been developed for the treatment of type 2 diabetes. Another class of drugs is based on an understanding of how these endogenous peptides are degraded in the body. Enzymes called dipeptidyl peptidase IV (DPP4) rapidly degrade endogenous GLP-1. Oral agents have been developed that inhibit DPP4 and, therefore, prolong the activity of endogenous GLP-1. There is a growing number of newer agents belonging to one of these two classes of drugs.

Examples of the former approach include Exenatide, Liraglutide and Lixisenatide, and there are numerous others in developments. Examples of the new class of drugs called DDP4 inhibitors include Sitagliptin, Saxagliptin, Linagliptin, Alogliptin and Vildagliptin. These are all currently available in the UK, and there are more in development.

GLP-1

Glucagon-like peptide-1 has the potential to improve glucose metabolism through a variety of different actions, as shown in Figure 20.1. Perhaps the most exciting is the suggested potential to improve beta cell insulin biosynthesis. They also inhibit secretion of glucagon, a somewhat neglected hormone in diabetes thus far. Figure 20.2 shows the impairment of the normal incretin response in patients with type 2 diabetes.

The incretin Exenatide is currently available in many countries, and a long-acting once-weekly preparation is also available. Liraglutide is a once-daily GLP-1 analogue and, more recently, Lixisenatide has become available. The use of these agents in type 2 diabetes is considered in chapter 7. Use of GLP-1 agonists do not preclude patients from driving. This is, therefore, particularly useful in patients whose occupation depends on driving public service vehicles. However, if adequate glycaemic control is not achieved with a GLP-1 agonist, then it is important to advise the patient that insulin is necessary.

When GLP-1 agonists are added to other oral agents, a further 11 mmol/mol reduction or so in HbA1c can be expected, although some patients may achieve more or less than this. A useful additional effect is weight loss, which is particularly helpful in overweight or obese type 2 patients. Excess risk of pancreatitis has been observed in post-marketing studies, although the absolute number of events is very small. It is, however, wise to avoid it in patients who may be otherwise at risk of pancreatitis. It must be used with caution along with insulin, as combination therapy has been shown to result in higher rates of hypoglycaemia. If prescribed with sulphonylureas it is important that, should hypoglycaemia occur, the dose of sulphonylurea is reduced.

DDP4 Inhibitors

As oral agents, these are a useful addition to metformin or sulphonylureas, as they appear to be relatively well tolerated. Sitagliptin was the first to become available in the UK, and is initially prescribed at a dose of 100 mg daily. Vildagliptin is available at a dose of 50 mg once or twice daily. They generally produce reductions of HbA1c between 7.7–11.0 mmol/mol, do not produce hypoglycaemia on their own and are weight-neutral. Linagliptin is used at a dose of 5 mg daily and does not need adjustment with renal impairment. These drugs are useful additional therapy, as they may produce further reduction in

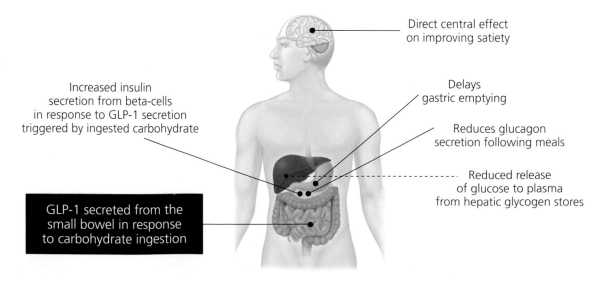

Direct central effect on improving satiety

Delays gastric emptying

Reduces glucagon secretion following meals

Reduced release of glucose to plasma from hepatic glycogen stores

Increased insulin secretion from beta-cells in response to GLP-1 secretion triggered by ingested carbohydrate

GLP-1 secreted from the small bowel in response to carbohydrate ingestion

Figure 20.1 Multiple effects of the incretin GLP-1 on glucose regulation.

The incretin effect: Response to oral vs IV glucose

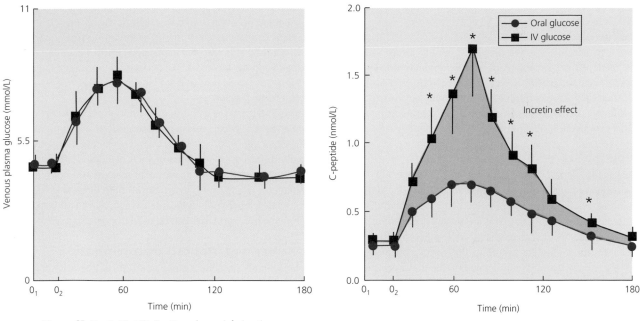

Mean ± SE; N = 6; *P ≤.05; O_1–O_2 = glucose infusion time.

The incretin effect: Is reduced in patients with type 2 diabetes

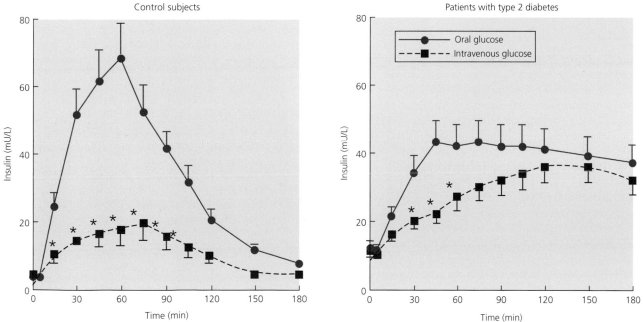

*P ≤.05 compared with respective value after oral load.

Figure 20.2 Endogenous insulin secretion (measured by C-peptide) responds more to oral than to intravenous glucose challenge due to the incretin effect. This effect is impaired in type 2 diabetes. Source: Nauck *et al.* (1986). Reproduced with permission of Springer Science+Business Media.

hyperglycaemia. There does not appear to be any change in cardiovascular risk with this class.

Obesity

Lifestyle modification is difficult once patients have type 2 diabetes. The disease itself, and the drugs often used by patients with diabetes, mean that progressive weight gain often occurs. Reduction in

weight using drug therapy brings with it benefits in terms of concomitant improvements in glycaemia, although these are often modest to the extent of about 5.5 mmol/mol of HbA1c reduction with orlistat.

These are useful additions to therapy for obese patients with type 2 diabetes. However, these drugs are ineffective, or their use is contra-indicated in many patients with obesity and diabetes. Therefore, there is a need for newer agents for obesity, especially if they have additional effects or added value in terms of improvement of associated risk factors, including diabetes.

Drugs for obesity

There is a paucity of effective drugs for obesity today and, after lifestyle management, the main effective treatment option available today is bariatric surgery, which is considered in Chapter 5. Orlistat, an intestinal fat absorption inhibitor, is the only anti-obesity drug available today, but GLP-1 agonists are in development for obesity and show promising results in trials.

SGLT inhibitors

Sodium/glucose linked transporter (SGLT) inhibitors, or SGLT2 inhibitors, are a new class of antihyperglycaemics introduced recently, which inhibit renal reabsorption of glucose by the proximal convoluted tubule. Some drugs in this class are already licensed for use and include dapagliflozin and canaglifolzin, while others are in development. These drugs eliminate some of the glucose normally reabsorbed by the kidney and do not depend on the presence of insulin. They are currently licensed for patients with type 2 diabetes and can be added onto any other medication, including insulin. Their use does not cause hypoglycaemia by itself, but doses of insulin or sulphonylurea may have to be adjusted. They are associated with some weight loss, but also with an increased incidence of urinary tract infections. Other SGLT1 inhibitors are in development.

The future

Glucocorticoid hormone pathways are being explored to produce new compounds that either inhibit their action or modulate their metabolism. 11β Hydroxysteroid dehydrogenase (11βHSD) type 1 enzyme inhibitors have potential to reverse central obesity and attendant complications. They are currently being subjected to trials. Other classes of drugs in development include bile acid sequestrants and G-protein coupled receptor-based drugs, for example GPR 40 and GPR119 agonists, which are still in the early stages of development.

Protein kinase C (PKC) inhibitors

Reducing the risk of complications in patients with diabetes is achieved mainly through control of blood glucose, blood pressure and dyslipidaemia. Clearly, this should be pursued with vigour to obtain the best control that can be achieved in the patient. Despite this, there are numerous patients whose glycaemic control remains poor. In such patients, there is potential for drug therapy to prevent the hyperglycaemia-induced damage on tissues that cause the complications. One such agent is a protein kinase C (PKC) inhibitor that has been developed recently. At the moment, ruboxistaurin remains in phase 3 development, as it requires further data to establish efficacy, although its safety appears to be quite good over a three-year period.

Artificial pancreas

Improvements in the technology of continuous monitoring and insulin delivery raise the prospect of a future 'artificial pancreas' through closure of the feedback loop between glucose measurements and insulin infusion rates. Work on such devices is actively under way but, at present, the monitoring technology is still not quite accurate enough for use in everyday situations. It is likely that this approach will be developed initially in intensively controlled hospital settings before the same principle can be used in portable devices.

Pancreas and islet cell transplantation

Whole-organ pancreas transplantation is possible, and has been particularly useful in patients also requiring kidney transplantation, as there is already a need for immunosuppressive therapy in such cases. Avoidance of the drawbacks of whole-organ donation is potentially possible by transplanting human islets of Langerhans, but this has proved extremely difficult due to aggressive, largely cell-mediated rejection responses in the host. These rejection mechanisms are more difficult to control than those following transplantation of heart, liver or kidney, for reasons that are still not well understood. Advances in this area will require these immunological barriers to be overcome, or may result from future stem cell technology.

Further reading and references

Deacon CF (2007). Incretin-based treatment of type 2 diabetes: glucagon-like peptide-1 receptor agonists and dipeptidyl peptidase-4 inhibitors. *Diabetes, Obesity and Metabolism* **9** (s1), 23–31.

Hovorka R (2005). Continuous glucose monitoring and closed loop systems. *Diabetic Medicine* **23**, 1–12.

Nauck M, Stöckmann F, Ebert R, Creutzfeldt W (1986). Reduced incretin effect in type 2 (non-insulin-dependent) diabetes. *Diabetologia* **29**(1), 46–52.

Jung PJ, Merrell RC (2006). Update on pancreatic islet cell transplantation. *Seminars in Surgical Oncology* **6**, 122–125.

Seaberg RM, Smukler SR, Kieffer TJ, *et al.* (2004). Clonal identification of multipotent precursors from adult mouse pancreas that generate neural and pancreatic lineages. *Nature Biotechnology* **22**, 1115–1124.

CHAPTER 21

Support for People Living with Diabetes

Tim Holt[1] and Sudhesh Kumar[2]

[1]Nuffield Department of Primary Care Health Sciences, Oxford University, UK
[2]Warwick Medical School, University of Warwick; and WISDEM, University Hospital, Coventry, UK

OVERVIEW

- Living with diabetes may be a personal issue, or may be an experience shared with an expanding global community.

- Accessing practical advice and support to help live with diabetes has become much easier due to web-based resources.

- A wide range of materials is available for patients, their carers and health professionals, for advice, education and advocacy.

- Support organisations also provide for those with no internet access, and those with physical barriers such as sensory impairments.

Introduction

A huge amount of help is available for people with diabetes, ranging from local groups offering individual support to international bodies advising patients, their carers and their health professionals (Figure 21.1). Advice and information needs to be tailored to the individual's needs and abilities but, provided sufficient time is taken, most patients can understand the basic principles of diabetes care and, of course, many become 'experts'. The Alphabet strategy, discussed earlier in this book, is as much about educating patients as it is about guiding clinicians on management. The Alphabet team have developed a range of readily accessible information sheets to assist in patient education (Figure 21.2). This gets the message across much more effectively than words alone.

Patient support organisations

For some, diabetes is a personal issue managed within a limited network of friends, family and health professionals while, for others, this network extends to the wider community and beyond. Diabetes can affect anyone at almost any age. Many find among this diversity a common thread of shared experience. For others, it is a very individual and private experience. Despite increasing public awareness of their needs, some people with diabetes may still feel isolated, stigmatised, discriminated against or otherwise in need of support and advocacy. Others may wish to share their success at overcoming personal goals. For all types of people, and for all those caring for them in any capacity, help is widely available. Over the last 20 years, the accessibility of health information has blurred the distinction between advice aimed at patients and that aimed towards health professionals, so that many of the organisations provide for all through a common point of access.

The websites of some major organisations are included in the 'Further reading' section at the end of this chapter. Familiarity with these resources is important for clinicians, who need to be able to advise patients on the most appropriate web resources, as many are available that are misleading. They may also need to direct patients to locally relevant information that is not always as clearly signposted.

Diabetes UK

This is the major charity representing and supporting people with diabetes and their carers in the UK.

Diabetes UK has nearly 300 volunteer support groups all over the UK to provide peer support at local as well as national level. Fundraising, campaigning, awareness raising and mutual support and advocacy are central activities, often taking place in social settings. The charity can help with practical issues, such as finding affordable health insurance that does not discriminate unfairly towards those with diabetes. The charity awards a prize for those who have lived with diabetes for over 50 years – an increasing number annually.

Balance, a magazine for people with diabetes, is published bi-monthly, and there are also regular e-newsletters keeping people up to date with what is going on in diabetes care. Many of the resources are available in different languages, and there is also CD- and audiotape-based information for those with visual impairment.

Diabetes UK also provides support for health professionals through policy statements, conferences, training materials, updates and research funding. It influences national policy as the major UK

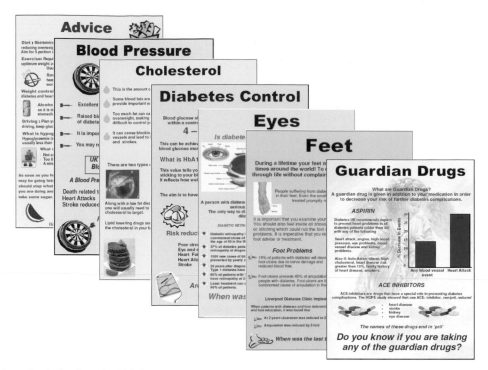

Figure 21.1 Patient information leaflets from the Alphabet team.

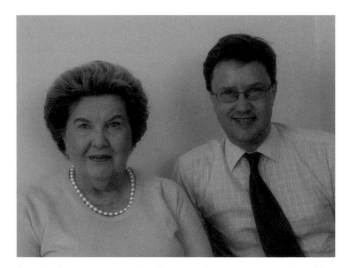

Figure 21.2 Seventy years on insulin: presenting as a seven-year-old with thirst and weight loss, this patient was started on insulin and rapidly regained her health. Pictured here with her current GP, Dr Tim Holt.

stakeholder representing users of diabetes services, and is consulted on policy development, including that of the National Institute for Health and Care Excellence (NICE). It holds an Annual Professional Conference and publishes a monthly professional journal, *Diabetic Medicine*. This journal is available free to those in the developing world, through the World Health Organization's HINARI programme. In addition, *Diabetes Update* is a quarterly journal on the latest news in diabetes.

The International Diabetes Federation (IDF)

The IDF applies similar principles to the worldwide community involved with diabetes, including patients, their carers and health professionals, and the research community. Their mission is 'to promote diabetes care, prevention and a cure worldwide'. They serve as an umbrella for national diabetes organisations all over the world. As well as its role in patient advocacy and education, the IDF has a strong academic role – for example, producing the IDF definition of the metabolic syndrome discussed in Chapter 4, which has become widely adopted.

The IDF's quarterly publication *Diabetes Voice*, published in English, French and Spanish, covers all aspects of diabetes care, education, prevention, research and practical aspects of living with diabetes.

The American Diabetes Association

While aimed at an American readership, the ADA's website contains lots of useful links that will be of interest to people in all countries, including those wishing to keep up with the latest research in diabetes. They also provide useful dietary advice (see Box 21.1) and recipes.

Patient.co.uk

The website www.patient.co.uk provides information both for patients and professionals on all sorts of health topics. Advantages of this resource are firstly its availability – it is linked to a major UK

Box 21.1 **Practical Advice on Healthy Eating from the American Diabetes Association Website**

- Eat lots of vegetables and fruits. Try picking from the rainbow of colours available to maximize variety. Eat non-starchy vegetables such as spinach, carrots, broccoli or green beans with meals.
- Choose whole grain foods over processed grain products. Try brown rice with your stir fry or whole wheat spaghetti with your favourite pasta sauce.
- Include dried beans (like kidney or pinto beans) and lentils into your meals.
- Include fish in your meals 2–3 times a week.
- Choose lean meats like cuts of beef and pork that end in 'loin', such as pork loin and sirloin.
- Remove the skin from chicken and turkey.
- Choose non-fat dairy such as skimmed milk, non-fat yogurt and non-fat cheese.
- Choose water and calorie-free 'diet' drinks instead of regular soda, fruit punch, sweet tea and other sugar-sweetened drinks.
- Choose liquid oils for cooking instead of solid fats that can be high in saturated and trans fats.
- Remember that fats are high in calories. If you're trying to lose weight, watch your portion sizes of added fats.
- Cut back on high-calorie snack foods and desserts like chips, cookies, cakes and full-fat ice cream.
- Eating too much of even healthful foods can lead to weight gain. Watch your portion sizes

clinical software system in primary care – and secondly that it provides the same advice to both patients and clinicians, but at two different levels. Patient UK articles and leaflets give a 'plain English' version, while 'Patient Plus' resources cover the issues in more depth. Both are available for patients as well as their professionals. All of the materials can be printed off during consultations or in the patient's home.

Summary

People living with diabetes have an increasing need to access support from local, national and global organisations offering practical advice, help and advocacy. Clinicians need to be able to signpost such people towards the most valuable resources, in order to maximise their benefits. Patient groups have an important role in funding diabetes research and in advising professional and governmental policy makers. They are an extremely active force in the battle to defeat diabetes.

Further reading

American Diabetes Association: www.diabetes.org
Diabetes UK: www.diabetes.org.uk
International Diabetes: Federation www.idf.org
Patient.co.uk: www.patient.co.uk
University of Oxford Diabetes Trials Unit: http://www.dtu.ox.ac.uk/

Index

abscess drainage 87
acanthosis nigricans 9
ACCORD Study 28, 40
acute painful neuropathies 92
age at diagnosis 2
albuminuria 30, 69
alcohol
    cardiovascular disease 31–33
    hypoglycaemia 52
    neuropathy 91, 93
    self-management of diabetes 56, 57
Alphabet Strategy 33
alpha-glucosidase inhibitors 38
alprostadil 93
American Diabetes Association (ADA)
    116–117
amputation 87–89, 110
anaemia 70
angiotensin-converting enzyme (ACE)
    inhibitors 28, 30–31, 70–72
angiotensin receptor blockers (ARB) 30, 71 72
animal insulins 47
Ankle Brachial Pressure Index (ABPI) 84
antibiotics 86–87
antidepressants 72
anti-vascular endothelial growth factor 78
apomorphine 93
artificial pancreas 114
ASCOT Study 32
aspirin 31, 71
autoantibodies 7–8
autonomic diarrhoea 92
autonomic neuropathy 92–93

background retinopathy 75–76
bariatric surgery 24–25
basal-bolus regimen 48
beta blockers 72
beta-cell function 16, 111
bezafibrate 72
biguanides 38
biphasic regimen 48

blood glucose *see* glycaemic control
blood pressure
    cardiovascular disease 28–30
    kidney disease 67–68
    living with diabetes 11–12
    pregnancy 101–102
    self-management of diabetes 56
    surveillance and follow-up 63–64
body mass index (BMI) 2, 23, 24, 63
breastfeeding 104–105
brittle diabetes 42

calcium channel blockers (CCB) 72
callus removal 86
carbohydrate 55–56, 59
cardiovascular disease (CVD) 27–34
    Alphabet Strategy 33
    blood pressure 28–30
    drug therapy 27–28, 30–32
    early detection and prevention 15–18
    glycaemic control 28–30
    life expectancy 27–28
    lifestyle 31–32
    lipids 31
    living with diabetes 11
    multifactorial interventions 32–33
    older patients 28
    polypharmacy 27
    renal impairment and albuminuria 30
    self-management of diabetes 55
CARDS Study 27, 29
cataract 80
Charcot's joint 83–85
childhood
    diagnosis 4
    hypoglycaemia 53
    insulin-resistant syndromes 9
    maturity onset diabetes in the young 8
    psychological issues 96
    type 2 diabetes 8, 15–16
    see also type 1 diabetes
cholesterol 12, 64

continuous glucose monitoring system
    (CGMS) 58–59
CoPilot program 60
coronary heart disease (CHD) 32–33
cotton wool spots 76

DAFNE programme 14, 42, 53, 60
debridement 87
depression
    kidney disease 72
    outcomes and assessment 97
    surveillance and follow-up 65
DESMOND 14
Diabetes Manual, The 14
Diabetes Prevention Program (DPP) 18, 24
Diabetes Register 107–108
Diabetes UK 115–116
diabetic foot 81–89
    callus removal 86
    Charcot's joint 83–85
    conservative management 86–87
    drug therapy 86–87
    infection 82, 85–88
    ischaemic and neuro-ischaemic foot 82–84,
        87–88
    maggot therapy 86–87
    management 84, 85–89
    neuropathy 81–82, 87–88
    patterns of presentation 82–83
    regular surveillance 83
    risk factors 81–82
    surgical intervention 87–89
    surveillance and follow-up 64–65, 83
    treatment of complications 85–86
    vascular insufficiency 81, 83
diabetic ketoacidosis (DKA) 41–43
    clinical features 41
    diagnosis 41–42
    early detection and prevention 41
    treatment 42–43
diabetic nephropathy *see* kidney disease
diabetic neuropathy *see* neuropathy